Also by George Foreman

By George
(with Joel Engel)

Also by Cherie Calbom

The Healthy Gourmet

Juicing for Life
(with Maureen Keane)

GEORGE FOREMAN'S
Knock-Out-the-Fat
Barbecue and Grilling Cookbook

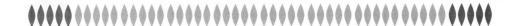

Villard
New York

GEORGE FOREMAN'S
Knock-Out-the-Fat
Barbecue and Grilling Cookbook

GEORGE FOREMAN
AND CHERIE CALBOM

Grateful acknowledgment is made to the following for permission to reprint
previously published material:

AVERY PUBLISHING GROUP: Two recipes from *The Sensuous Vegetarian Barbecue*
by Vicki Rae Chelf and Dominique Biscotti. Copyright © 1994.
Published by Avery Publishing Group, Garden City Park, New York.
Reprinted by permission.

CLARKSON N. POTTER/PUBLISHERS: Three recipes from *The Healthy Gourmet*
by Cherie Calbom. Copyright © 1996 by Cherie Calbom, M.S.
Reprinted by permission of Clarkson N. Potter/Publishers, a member
of the Crown Publishing Group.

Library of Congress Cataloging-in-Publication Data
Foreman, George.
George Foreman's knock-out-the-fat barbecue and grilling cookbook /
by George Foreman and Cherie Calbom.—1st ed.
p.   cm.
ISBN 0-679-77149-2
1. Barbecue cookery.   2. Low-fat diet—Recipes.   I. Calbom,
Cherie.   II. Title.
TX840.B3F67   1996
641.5'784—dc20   96-6020

Printed in the United States of America on acid-free paper
89

Book design by Deborah Kerner

To my mother,
Nancy R. Foreman,
who year after year
took small amounts of meat and vegetables
and turned them into meals
fit for a king.
—GEORGE FOREMAN

To my father-in-law,
John E. Calbom, Sr.,
who fired up the grill
for the last time this year
and left us August 11, 1995, to plead our cases
in the courts of heaven.
—CHERIE CALBOM

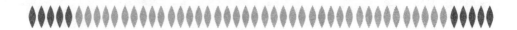

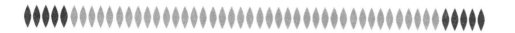

PREFACE

DURING MY BOXING CAREER, I HAVE HAD MORE THAN ONE HUNdred KOs. I admit that if a fight goes the distance, I'm disappointed, regardless of whether I get the decision. I like knockouts—I don't go for the points; I go for the big win. I feel the same way about eating the right foods. I go for the big winners: those foods that provide the best nourishment for my body. The recipes in this book illustrate the way I like to eat, highlighting the very foods I enjoy most now that I am taking extra-good care of myself. They're all big winners and, I'm proud to say, they knock out the fat!

My eating habits have changed significantly over the years. Today, I understand the value of a diet that's low in fat and includes plenty of vegetables, fruits, pasta, rice, bread, fish, and chicken. Red meat—which used to represent *good* eating to me—is low on the list. I still indulge in it, but only now and then.

This book gives me the opportunity to share my revelations about eating well and eating right: the most important one being that the food I eat now tastes great! I have never enjoyed eating more than I do now. I still like sizable portions and full-flavored, juicy food—when you're my size and work out as diligently as I do, you need lots of good food to keep going. Cherie Calbom, a nutritionist and top-notch cook who developed the recipes on the following pages, wanted to make them healthy and nutritious. I told her, "George wants taste! George wants juicy!" And as I tasted the dishes she prepared, following my dietary preferences and beliefs, one word leaped from my mouth over and over again: "Wow!"

There are two secrets to the success of these recipes: The first is proper preparation, good seasoning, and careful cooking; the second is using nutritious ingredients and lowering the fat.

As a boxer, I know that fat slows you down. I remember only too well when I weighed in at more than 315 pounds. I had been eating with great gusto and little thought from 1977, when I left boxing, until 1987, when I decided that the time had come to return to what I did best. I had ballooned almost beyond recognition. I needed my body back! And so I set about learning how to eat correctly as well as devising (and sticking to) a grueling workout schedule. Like anything you set your mind to, both the food and the exercise worked.

When I was boxing in the 1960s and '70s, I ate mostly steak and big salads. That was classic training-table fare. I was young and in excellent shape, able to win fights with a first-round knockout. I won the heavyweight gold medal for boxing at the 1968 Olympics, and went on to become heavyweight champion of the world. In those days I hardly considered what I ate as long as I had enough! And believe me, only *a lot* of food was enough for George Foreman.

But I know now that the foods I ate then are not the right foods to sustain my body for a lifetime. The human body needs to be nourished without contributing to obesity, high blood pressure, high cholesterol, and other "silent" health problems that can cause disease later in life. Just as we strive for a good job, a family, a nice home, and a savings account, we should strive for a healthy body. Who doesn't want to live a long and healthy life? But it takes planning.

That's why I wrote this book with nutritionist Cherie Calbom. The recipes, cooking techniques, and nutritional information will help you plan your own diet so that you, too, can feel better and nourish your body properly. You may have to alter your priorities so that you can eat less red meat and more vegetables and fruit, but take it from me: It's worth it!

As you will discover on the following pages, my journey from boyhood to being a world-class athlete who paid no attention *whatsoever* to what he ate to being a forty-seven-year-old heavyweight champion of the world who is still in great shape was a long one. But I learned so much along the way about the value of good food, proper nutrition, and regular exercise that I want to pass some of it on to you, along with some new tips I've learned from Cherie.

I hope you enjoy the recipes contained here. Every single one has my personal seal of approval. Each one is a winner. Once you begin eating better and taking care of yourself, I promise you will feel like a champion—just like I do!

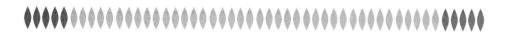

ACKNOWLEDGMENTS

WE WISH TO EXPRESS OUR DEEP AND LASTING APPRECIATION TO the people who have assisted us with this book, especially Chef Mark Evans, whose creative ideas and culinary skills took our recipes to new levels of flavor and taste.

A sincere thank-you to Steven Sapienza, R.D., of Nutritional Analysis Consultants, in Livonia, Michigan, for his expert nutritional analysis and quick response to our needs.

Our hearty thanks to Mary Goodbody for her creative writing skills and timely work.

Many thanks to Cherie's husband, John, our "official taste-tester," who made suggestions and approved of and thoroughly enjoyed every recipe in this book.

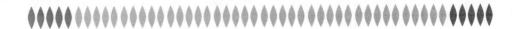

CONTENTS

Preface ≈ ix

Acknowledgments ≈ xi

Introduction ≈ 3

CHAPTER ONE: Eating to Win ≈ 9

CHAPTER TWO: Grilling and Barbecuing in Healthful Style ≈ 20

CHAPTER THREE: Facts About Grills and Grilling ≈ 25

CHAPTER FOUR: Marinades ≈ 33

CHAPTER FIVE: Dry Rubs ≈ 37

CHAPTER SIX: Barbecue Sauces ≈ 42

CHAPTER SEVEN: Burgers and Sandwiches ≈ 47

CHAPTER EIGHT: Beef ≈ 63

CHAPTER NINE: Fish and Seafood ≈ 78

CHAPTER TEN: Lamb ≈ 99

CHAPTER ELEVEN: Poultry ≈ 112

CHAPTER TWELVE: Pork ≈ 138

CHAPTER THIRTEEN: Vegetables and Vegetarian Barbecue ≈ 153

Glossary of Terms and Ingredients ≈ 165

Index ≈ 169

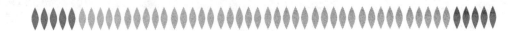

GEORGE FOREMAN'S
Knock-Out-the-Fat
Barbecue and Grilling Cookbook

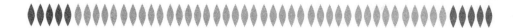

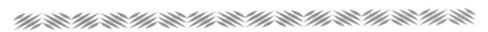

INTRODUCTION

Getting Off to a Good Start

I CANNOT DENY THAT MANY PEOPLE TOLD ME I WAS NUTS when I decided to return to the ring after a ten-year retirement. I weighed more than 300 pounds and was out of shape, to say the least. I had gained so much weight in part because, shortly after hanging up my gloves, I discovered fast-food restaurants. I found enormous pleasure in driving up and down the highways in my native Texas, stopping at every hamburger, barbecue, pizza, and taco joint along the way. When I had been fighting, I was barely aware of the existence of these emporiums. Now they seemed to be everywhere I turned, and I just loved that grease and fat. I often topped off one of these frequent binges with a double-scoop ice-cream cone.

But in 1986 I decided to get back into shape. The first thing I did was organize an intense exercise program for myself. I understood how to do this—I was an athlete. I ran for miles, many more than I ever had before. When I couldn't go outside to work out, I used the treadmill. I skipped backward around the perimeter of the ring. I jumped rope. I punched the heavy bag for 30 minutes with nothing but right hands, followed by 30 minutes of left hands and another 30 minutes of jabs. Despite all this training, I couldn't break the 300-pound mark on the scale. What was wrong? Maybe it was my diet, something I had paid little attention to and understood less. A friend suggested I start eating pasta and other complex carbohydrates rather than beef. It worked like a charm, and in time I reached 230 pounds. All right!

Staying with Good Habits

Over the last eight or nine years, I have come to appreciate food that's prepared simply and well. I understand the concept of eating for energy, for a long life, and to win—as well as for great taste. I have learned to trim the fat from meat and poultry before cooking them—and this includes removing chicken skin. I have developed a fondness for fish and vegetables. My favorite fish is catfish—and I prefer it pan-fried or deep-fried—but I also like other fish. For example, I am fond of swordfish, which is great for grilling because it holds up over the intense heat, staying firm and meaty.

I have learned that a strictly vegetarian diet does not suit me as a permanent thing. However, I will go for an entire month eating nothing but vegetables to keep my weight down and my strength up. When I was growing up, I rarely ate meat. We were too poor to afford it more than once in a blue moon, and so, without actually realizing it, I ate a lot of vegetarian meals that my mother put on the table. I grew up big and strong. The vegetables worked! I replicate that diet two or three times every year for about a month at a time, eating nothing but vegetables, with some fruit, bread, rice, and pasta tossed in for good measure. I truly believe this diet contributes to my strength and well-being.

When I end one of these vegetable-intensive months, I happily return to eating meat and fish. Undeniably, beef is my favorite as far as flavor, and I usually go right out and grab a steak. But I know that, as an athlete and someone who cares about his health, I can't eat beef too often. I also find that the weight I put on when I eat beef is far more difficult to shed than the weight I might gain from a diet of vegetables, chicken, and fish. My list of most-often-consumed proteins begins with fish, followed by chicken and lamb, with beef and pork trailing far behind.

Cravings and Indulgences

I can't deny that I love the flavor of red meat. For me, nothing beats a well-cooked cheeseburger fairly dripping with melted cheese. Who ever thought of this combination? I know it's not a healthful one, but it sure tastes good. When I was a kid growing up in Houston, I was obsessed with getting enough to eat. Occasionally I got hold of a quarter and I'd use it to buy a hamburger. I could rarely afford the extra nickel for the cheese—although I would crave it every time. Maybe this is why I like cheeseburgers so much today: They represent the ultimate luxury.

When I crave meat, I think it's a way that my body communicates with me. "Hey, man, you need some more protein," my body says. "You're working out really hard, your supplements are down, and you're going to have to get more vitamins." At this point, I might make a trip to the health food store and question the folks there about protein supplements and the vitamins I need. I'm always learning something new about how nutrients work and how our bodies metabolize them. But if I'm no more than ten or fifteen pounds over my fighting weight when I crave protein, I usually treat myself to a cheeseburger. But just one!

I also like pork sausage. Nothing pleases me more than using my electric grill first thing in the morning and cooking breakfast sausage patties for my kids and me. As they grill, the fat just seems to disappear. And when the sausage is done, it's just delicious. I remember as a child being rationed to one piece of bacon on the Sundays when my mother could afford it. The smell of the bacon cooking was absolutely tantalizing, and the single rasher hardly satisfied. On more than one occasion, my beseeching gaze convinced my mother to sacrifice her piece for me. Oh, how I appreciate that extra bit of bacon even to this day, and I still consider bacon a treat.

Growing Up Poor

Although we didn't discuss it in our house, the Foremans were poor. I was one of seven children, raised by my mother in the area of Houston called the Fifth Ward. I spent much of my childhood and youth being hungry. My mother, Nancy Ree Foreman, worked seven days a week scraping together enough money to sustain her children and herself, but it was not enough to provide us with more than the bare basics. For a boy who was destined to be six feet four inches and big-boned, the amount of food seemed inadequate. My poor mother asked herself over and over, "How in the world do you fill up a boy like George Foreman?" But somehow she managed to keep me going, and I grew into a strong and healthy young man. I will always be grateful for her care and love—they got me through the hard times more surely than any meal.

Poor or not, we celebrated with good food on holidays. I still remember my mother's sweet potato pie on Thanksgiving, along with her baked ham. She and my aunts prepared rice in special ways on holidays, too, so that it became as much a centerpiece of the meal as the meat—and went a lot further, too. (I now realize this was for economic reasons as well as to feed us.)

Although I dropped out of school in junior high, I got a "second chance" when I signed up for the Job Corps, a program developed during the Johnson administration as part of the president's War on Poverty. I traveled from Houston to a Job Corps training center in Oregon—a trip that first opened my eyes to the world beyond Texas. (I had never before been on a plane and was thrilled that I could eat two lunches!) I attribute my success in life in large part to the Job Corps. It gave me an education, vocational training, and, most important, a sense of self-respect. During my time with the corps, I began boxing. The rest, as they say, is history.

I do want to mention a kindness I will never forget. Mrs. Moon, the cook at the Oregon training center, took an interest in me, and I was thrilled (and a little nervous) when she invited me home with her for a weekend meal with her family. I vividly remember the meal she prepared. Not only was there pot roast, potatoes, vegetables, and bread, there was enough for George Foreman to have seconds—several times! I visited with her and her family a number of times after that, but that first meal remains most firmly lodged in my memory.

Memorable Meals

While I remember the pot roast I shared with Mrs. Moon and her family, it is not the only meal that stays in my memory. The one that meant the very most was the meal my wife, Joan, prepared shortly after we were married. I had spent some months insisting she learn how to cook my "favorites" just like my mother had made them. Joan was willing and happy to please me, but one day I arrived home to the aroma of an unfamiliar dish coming from the grill. What's this? I wondered. Lamb with potatoes. The absolute *best* lamb and potatoes I had ever put in my mouth! From that day on, my favorites included dishes Joan created.

I can't imagine a more perfect meal than one shared with my family. My wife and I love having all nine of our children sitting around the table with us. A big, juicy turkey in the middle of the table is just right for this crowd. I appreciate having the right fork for salad, the right spoon for soup, and so forth. I have made sure all my children have good table manners, as it makes the dining experience much more pleasant and makes everyone feel welcome at the meal. In return, I make sure there is enough food on the table. When you've grown up poor, you really appreciate having enough to eat. And since I have learned so much about proper nutrition, I always try to have a good balance of healthy foods on the table. Not too much meat, not too many vegeta-

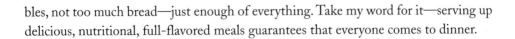
bles, not too much bread—just enough of everything. Take my word for it—serving up delicious, nutritional, full-flavored meals guarantees that everyone comes to dinner.

Why I Wrote This Book

Food is plentiful in this great country. There are vast, rolling fields planted with grains, which are fed to chickens, cattle, and hogs. We also mill the grains into flour for wonderful breads and other baked goods. We grow all sorts of vegetables, legumes, and fruits. Seas, lakes, and streams are stocked with fish and seafood. But our landscape is also dotted with fast-food restaurants, shops selling ice cream in "designer" flavors, and supermarkets and convenience stores selling packaged high-fat snacks. With all this bounty, it's not surprising that as a nation we tend to overeat. Too much of our food is loaded with fat—and Americans have bought into the old saying that "fat gives taste, fat gives juice." This may be true, but it is not the whole truth. A little fat goes a long way, and many other ingredients make foods tasty and juicy as well. Cooking techniques contribute greatly to how food tastes, too.

The recipes that Cherie and I have assembled are meant for grilling or barbecuing, two of the best ways to prepare meals without added fat. When you grill, the food cooks over direct heat and the fat melts and drips away. There is no need to add oil or butter—which other books tell you to use to prevent food from sticking to the pan. Relying on grilling means that if you begin with a piece of fish, meat, or poultry trimmed of visible fat, you will end up with even less fat than you started with. I call that KO-ing the fat!

But, you may argue, fat is an indisputable agent for transferring flavor. That's true, but it is not the *only* one, nor does it have to be used in great quantity. Cherie and I use marinades, dry rubs, and sauces to add zest, seal in natural juices, and accentuate flavors. Try our Lean Mean Steak Fajitas (page 74) or Texas Barbecued Beef Ribs (page 76) to get an idea of how to cook without much fat and without sacrificing any flavor.

There are also a number of recipes for some of my old favorites—George's Powerburger (page 48) and the Foreman Family Breakfast Sausage (page 140), to name just two—as well as for some new favorites: Grilled Turkey Cutlets with Honey-Dijon-Rosemary Marinade (page 134) and Ginger-Lime Swordfish (page 83). Lots of fish, lots of chicken and turkey, plenty of vegetables—and some lamb, beef, and pork. That's how I *like* to eat, *know* I should eat, and *plan* to eat for the rest of my life.

I grew up wanting more food than my mother could afford. Once I achieved success and could eat as much as I wanted, I did not understand how *what* I put in my mouth affected my overall health. As I approached my forties and started paying attention to my body so that I could resume my boxing career, I came to understand that the "old" George Foreman was never going to enter the ring again—not with the same attitude and abilities he had in the 1960s and '70s. The person who would step into the spotlight would be the "new" George Foreman, with very different attitudes, training habits, and eating habits. This does not mean I don't still love food. I will always like to eat! I am pleased to have this opportunity to show you what I like to eat, and to explain why it is important to pay attention to your daily diet. Whether we are athletes or not, we all have to eat right to be champs.

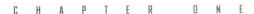

EATING TO WIN

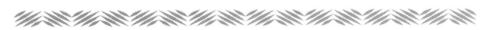

Y OU DON'T HAVE TO BE IN TRAINING FOR THE HEAVYWEIGHT boxing championship of the world to benefit from eating healthier. Everyone wins by eating right. You can help prevent heart disease, cancer, and many other degenerative diseases by following a healthy diet. You can maintain your desired weight and a physically fit body. By eating right you *will* promote a stronger immune system and thus suffer fewer colds and flu. And you will look healthier, with brighter eyes, shinier hair, and a better complexion. The old adage is true: "We are what we eat."

So what does it mean to eat right? Everyone has an opinion. There are all sorts of food fads. Currently, the focus is on getting the fat out of our diet. That's a good thing. No one is contesting the fact that Americans eat too much fat, and we know that excess fat contributes to a variety of physical problems—from obesity to heart disease. That's why Cherie and I have reduced the fat in our recipes wherever possible to create dishes that are not only healthier but tasty, too.

The Facts About Fat

Overconsumption of fat contributes to obesity, cancer, heart and artery disease, and a host of other physical ills, so it makes good sense to limit our intake of dietary fat and cholesterol. Many health-conscious consumer organizations recommend this, but diet surveys indicate that people are still eating about 40 to 50 percent of their calories as fat—more than our forefathers ate at the turn of the century, and far more than we need with our sedentary lifestyles.

There is more than double the number of calories in a gram of fat versus a gram of protein or carbohydrate: 1 gram of fat equals 9 calories, compared to 1 gram of protein or carbohydrate, which contains 4 calories. Fat is a concentrated form of energy that's stored by the body, not eliminated. That's why, when fat is eaten in excess, it really puts on the weight. Too much stored fat makes people obese and, over time, undermines their health.

All of us need to limit the amount of fat in our diet (especially saturated fat) if we want to maintain a trim weight and sustain a healthy body. Our cookbook focuses on some of the most fatty foods we can eat, namely animal products. But there are a number of things we can do to reduce the fat content of those foods and their accompaniments. Specifically, we can take the skin off chicken and turkey before cooking them. We can eat less red meat, butter, margarine, cheese, cream, mayonnaise, fat-rich desserts, junk food, and fast food. And we can eat a high-fiber diet consisting of plenty of vegetables, whole grains, and legumes. The following pages show you how you can "knock the fat out of your diet before it knocks the life out of you!"

We both have a word of caution, however. In the furor to avoid all fats, too often people substitute imitation foods for the real thing just because the label says *fat-free* or *fat-reduced.* Imitation, chemical-laden products are not necessarily going to promote better health. In most cases, these are products with molecular changes that the body can't handle or doesn't know how to eliminate, and over time they can contribute to poor health. For example, it is far better to eat butter rather than margarine. Margarine is loaded with *trans fatty acids,* unhealthy substances that are created in the process of making the margarine. Research has shown that trans fats, abundant in most margarines, are detrimental to our health. Then there are the new "fake fats" that give the impression you can devour bags of chips, for example, with no ill effects. No one knows what these new fats will do to the body, although many health professionals have serious concerns. Stick with *real* food, and that means even real fat—fat found in nature. *But* eat it only occasionally and in small portions.

The Fats of Life

With all the attention on fat as the dietary villain of the decade, we couldn't complete this section without mentioning that some fats have been given a bum rap.

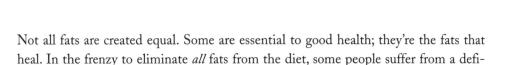

Not all fats are created equal. Some are essential to good health; they're the fats that heal. In the frenzy to eliminate *all* fats from the diet, some people suffer from a deficiency of essential fatty acids.

The true heroes of the fat world are the omega fatty acids, omega-3 and omega-6. Although all fatty acids produce 9 calories of energy per gram, all are not used the same. The body likes to use unsaturated and essential fatty acids for important functions. It saves the omega-3s and omega-6s for vital hormonelike functions. These fatty acids are also key nutrients in the most active tissues, those of the brain, sense organs, adrenal glands, and testes.

Scientific studies have shown that omega-3s, which are abundant in fatty cold-water fish, actually reduce the risk of heart disease and some cancers. They also can halt inflammation caused by autoimmune diseases such as rheumatoid arthritis. Omega-3 consumption today has decreased to about one sixth the level existing in our diet in the mid-1800s, while omega-6 consumption has doubled. The ratio of omega-3 to omega-6 fatty acids should be about 2:1. For this reason we recommend that your first choice in animal proteins be fish.

Two of the omega-3s are eicosapentaenoic acid (EPA) and docosahexaenoic acid (DHA), which are found in the oils of cold-water fish like salmon, trout, mackerel, and sardines, and in smaller amounts in other fish. The omega-3s are abundant in more than fish, however. Alpha linoleic acid (omega-3) is found in flax, hemp, canola, and soy bean oils and dark green leafy vegetables.

Linoleic acid and gamma-linoleic acid (GLA) are the omega-6 fatty acids. Linoleic acid is found in safflower, sunflower, soybean, walnut, pumpkin, sesame, and flax oils. Borage, black currant seed oil, and evening primrose oil are the best sources of GLA.

When we talk about fats in relation to a healthy body, it should not be assumed that we have to avoid them altogether. We need to eat them in the right balance: not too little, not too much—and enough of the healthy kind. No more than 30 percent of our daily calories should come from fat. Out of that number, no more than 10 percent should come from saturated fat (mainly found in animal products), with no more than 300 mg of cholesterol daily. The remaining 20 percent of calories from fat should come from unsaturated and essential fatty acids, with emphasis on the omega-3s: fish—especially fatty cold-water fish—dark green leafy vegetables, and canola, flax, and soybean oils.

Healthy Eating Made Simple

It is quite easy to learn how to balance animal proteins with other food groups to create a nourishing eating plan for you and your family. Lowering the fat in your diet is a very good idea, but it's not the only thing that contributes to good health.

To better understand what it means to eat healthy, let's look at the Food Guide Pyramid introduced by the U.S. Department of Agriculture (USDA) in 1991. This helpful graphic (see page 13) has replaced the outdated Four Food Groups many of us learned about in school. This guide shows that bread and cereal grains, which form the base of the pyramid, should likewise form the base of a healthful diet. Vegetables and fruit are on the tier just above and, as most of us know, should be increased in our diet. Dairy products, meat, poultry, fish, eggs, dry beans, and nuts share the third level; these foods should be eaten in smaller quantities than many of us are accustomed to doing. Finally, at the very top are fats, oils, and sweets—foods that we should eat very sparingly.

Not only does the pyramid show which foods are the most important to good nutrition, it clearly indicates how much of them should be eaten in relation to other foods, as a percentage of overall caloric intake. As a general rule of thumb, healthy, active men need 2,200 to 2,800 calories per day; women need about 1,600 to 2,000 calories daily, depending on activity; and children and teens need 1,200 to 2,200 calories each day. The following sections describe the principal food groups and give the number of servings recommended for each group.

Bread, Cereal, Rice, and Pasta

This bottom level of the pyramid represents the most important food group. Within this group, the healthiest choices are *whole* grains (unprocessed grains that contain the germ and bran) such as are found in whole-grain cereal, whole-grain bread, whole-grain pasta, and brown rice. The USDA recommends 6 to 11 servings of this food group each day. While it may be hard to eat that much every day, obviously the greatest emphasis should be placed on these foods. A single serving is 1 slice of bread, $^1/_2$ cup cooked rice or pasta, $^1/_2$ cup cooked cereal, or 1 ounce ready-to-eat cereal.

Vegetables

Although the Food Guide Pyramid recommends 3 to 5 servings of this group a day, you can benefit by eating even more. Vegetables are among the richest sources of vitamins, minerals, enzymes, antioxidants, and phytonutrients (*phyto* means plant).

FOOD GUIDE PYRAMID

A Guide to Daily Food Choices

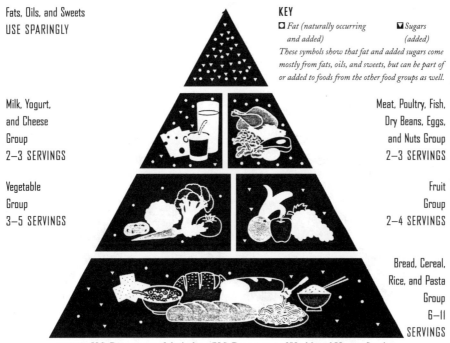

Fats, Oils, and Sweets
USE SPARINGLY

KEY
◻ *Fat (naturally occurring and added)*   ◼ *Sugars (added)*
These symbols show that fat and added sugars come mostly from fats, oils, and sweets, but can be part of or added to foods from the other food groups as well.

Milk, Yogurt,
and Cheese
Group
2–3 SERVINGS

Meat, Poultry, Fish,
Dry Beans, Eggs,
and Nuts Group
2–3 SERVINGS

Vegetable
Group
3–5 SERVINGS

Fruit
Group
2–4 SERVINGS

Bread, Cereal,
Rice, and Pasta
Group
6–11
SERVINGS

SOURCE: *U.S. Department of Agriculture/U.S. Department of Health and Human Services*

Use the Food Guide Pyramid to help you eat better every day . . . the Dietary Guidelines way. Start with plenty of Breads, Cereals, Rice, and Pasta; Vegetables; and Fruits. Add two to three servings from the Milk group and two to three servings from the Meat group. Each of these food groups provides some, but not all, of the nutrients you need. No one food group is more important than another—for good health you need them all. Go easy on fats, oils, and sweets, the foods in the small tip of the pyramid.

Lightly steam a variety of vegetables, include them with meat, poultry, or seafood on skewers for healthier kabobs, and add them to stuffings, sauces, soups, stews, casseroles, frittatas, and pizzas. Have a fresh salad at least once a day. Cut up vegetable sticks and keep them on hand for quick snacks. A single serving is $1/2$ cup chopped raw or cooked vegetables, 1 cup leafy raw vegetables, or $3/4$ cup vegetable juice.

Fruits

With their appealing, sweet taste, fruits are easy to include regularly in our diet. The USDA recommends 2 to 4 servings a day, which should be very simple to accomplish, especially if fresh juices are included. (Cherie and I don't recommend canned or bottled juice.) One exception to this serving recommendation is for people who suffer from sugar metabolism problems—hypoglycemia or diabetes. If you have either of these conditions, unless otherwise advised by a health professional, you should limit your fruit intake to 1 serving a day, while increasing your vegetable servings. A single serving is 1 piece of fruit or melon wedge, $3/4$ cup fruit juice, $1/2$ cup canned fruit, or $1/4$ cup dried fruit.

Meat, Poultry, Fish, Dried Beans, Eggs, and Nuts

Only 10 to 15 percent of your daily calories should come from proteins, so it is advisable to include no more than 3 ounces of cooked meat, poultry, or fish in a serving, and no more than 2 to 3 servings per day. Proteins from animals are the highest in fat, cholesterol, and calories, and therefore should be consumed in small amounts. Nuts and seeds are also high in fat and should be limited, especially when you are watching calories. However, the oils in nuts are not saturated and they are cholesterol-free. Legumes, such as dried beans, lentils, and split peas, are the lowest in fat, contain no cholesterol, and are smart protein choices. A single serving is $2^{1}/_{2}$ to 3 ounces of cooked lean meat, poultry, or fish; $1/2$ cup cooked beans, lentils, or split peas; 1 egg; 2 tablespoons peanut butter; or $1/4$ cup seeds or nuts.

Milk, Yogurt, and Cheese

Consumption of dairy products is encouraged because of their calcium content. Two to three servings a day are recommended by the USDA. However, due to their higher fat and cholesterol content and because some people are allergic to dairy products or suffer respiratory congestion when they eat them, it is important to note that other calcium-rich foods can be substituted, such as dark leafy greens, corn tortillas made with lime, soy products, seeds, and nuts. (If you omit servings of dairy products, be sure to include 2 or 3 servings of other calcium-rich foods.) A single serving is 1 cup of milk or yogurt, $\frac{1}{2}$ cup cottage cheese, or $1\frac{1}{2}$ to 2 ounces cheese.

Fats, Oils, and Sweets

These foods represent the small tip of the pyramid and should be used sparingly. The USDA gives no recommended daily servings. You should strive to eat fewer servings of these foods than of those from any other group. This category includes salad dressings, cream, butter, margarine, sugars, soft drinks, candies, and sweet desserts. Alcoholic beverages are also part of this group. Fats, oils, and sweets provide calories but very few vitamins and minerals. A single serving is 1 tablespoon butter, margarine, or oil; 2 tablespoons salad dressing; or 4 tablespoons syrup or sugar.

The Right Food Plan for You

Though the Food Guide Pyramid is a good general nutrition guide, we also want to point out that it is a springboard from which to design an eating plan that is right for your particular nutritional needs. People are all different. Just as they have different physical features, height, and bone structure, they also have unique metabolic differences, which means that they react very differently to a variety of foods. Take, for example, the first tier of the pyramid and the recommendation of 6 to 11 servings of grains each day. Not everyone does well eating lots of carbohydrates throughout the day. Some people become sleepy and lethargic if they consume too many of these foods during the day. They would do much better eating the major portion of their grains in the evening, when getting sleepy is welcomed. Cherie does best taking in most of her carbohydrates at dinner, and with the exception of having whole-grain cereal for breakfast, she feels the most alert and energetic during the day if she eats vegetables and legumes (beans, lentils, or split peas) or animal protein for lunch. The same goes for fruit. When the eat-only-fruit-until-noon craze came along, again Cherie was one who was nearly asleep by 10 A.M. after an all-fruit breakfast.

One thing is for certain—no one does well on a diet that is largely composed of high-fat animal proteins or fat-rich junk food. Today, most athletes and health-conscious Americans eat more complex carbohydrates, such as pasta and brown rice, legumes, and lots of vegetables, with fresh fruit for snacks and dessert, and they limit their intake of animal proteins.

When I returned to boxing at the age of thirty-seven, after ten years away from competition, I quickly learned that the dietary rules had changed since the 1970s. Steak was no longer considered smart nutrition for an athlete. Athletes who were serious about training were eating plenty of vegetables and whole grains and smaller amounts of animal proteins. I discovered that the fat I put on from eating meat was very hard to take off. To reach my desired weight, I had to cut out red meat and fast food. Even though I joke about cheeseburgers, I now only eat them occasionally.

The right diet for me was more like the one I ate while living with my mom. As I thought about the foods my mother cooked and served me, I realized that I could attribute my physical strength to all the vegetables I ate while searching for the few pieces of meat in the stew, along with the bread to fill myself up. Today, when I really want to keep my body going strong, I stay away from animal products for a while, sometimes for up to a month at a time, and I eat lots and lots of vegetables with pasta and whole grains. When I choose animal proteins, especially when I'm in training, it's often fish—catfish and swordfish are my favorites.

It is important to learn how to listen to your body and the feedback it sends. Ask yourself some important questions: Are the foods you're eating contributing to a trim, physically fit body, or are you constantly struggling with a weight problem? After eating certain foods do you feel happy, energetic, strong, confident, and mentally alert? Do certain foods make you feel fatigued, depressed, lethargic, agitated, or mentally fogged in? Look for physical reactions and signs. What are some of your immediate responses to what you eat? Do you have any ongoing physical problems and could they be diet related? Take inventory of how you feel one or two days after eating certain foods. And look at your fitness level and how you generally feel from week to week.

The Diet for Champs

Eating to win definitely means cutting the fat, and Cherie and I have done our best to knock it out of the dishes we've created. For starters, grilling is a much healthier way to cook meat, poultry, and fish than pan-frying or deep-frying is, because the fat drips off. Grilling is even healthier than baking, where the food sits in some fat, or broiling, where a little fat remains on the broiling pan. When meat sits in fat, it reabsorbs some of it. When food is grilled, the fat constantly drips off.

To help you cut the fat even more, we offer several fat-free marinades. When we do use oil, it's canola oil (which is monounsaturated) or olive oil (known for its health benefits), and we use very little butter. Skin is always removed from poultry. Lean cuts of meat are recommended as often as possible. In an attempt to make the recipes healthier, we've used no refined sugars; only honey, pure maple syrup, or black-strap molasses are added for sweetness. Fresh ingredients are our first choice whenever possible. And naturally grown meats and poultry and organically grown fruits and vegetables are our first recommendation.

We also caution you not to get so caught up in the fat furor that you think just reducing your intake of fat is going to prevent all sorts of ills. Though keeping your weight at a healthy level is an excellent start, it's not the total answer. Eating to win also means eating the right balance of healthful foods. Vegetables, whole grains, legumes, and fresh fruit should form the largest part of your daily diet. For the best nutrition some of the vegetables and fruit should be raw, and choose *organic* produce (foods grown without pesticides or herbicides) whenever possible. Eat fish two or three times per week for additional protein and omega-3 fatty acids. Opt for poultry instead of red meat. And choose red meat (lamb, beef, or pork) only as an occasional indulgence. Reach for fresh fruit for snacks and dessert. And follow me, the champ, by cutting out fast food and junk food, eating them only on rare occasions.

Listen to your body's responses to what you eat and when you eat certain foods. You can reap physical rewards in so doing. Like Cherie and me, you should benefit from occasional vegetarian days, whether it's a day or two a week or an occasional week or month during the year.

When judging your fat intake, we recommend looking at your food choices on a more realistic week-by-week basis rather than analyzing each meal, which could quickly drive you to frustration. If, for example, you decide to have the thick, juicy Stuffed Pork Chops with Honey-Pineapple Marinade (page 141) or the Country-Style Ribs with Louisiana Bacon Barbecue Sauce (page 145) one night, you could make the next day's dinner a fish meal and prepare the Orange Roughy with Zesty Fat-Free Marinade (page 88). You could also cut your fat intake for the week by having one vegetarian day. Try Garden Burgers (page 61) for a pleasant surprise.

By following the suggestions in this cookbook, you can be eating healthier every day. If you want to win the prize of good health, it's worth every bit of effort that you make. With just a little planning, the knowledge of what foods to choose, delicious recipes from our cookbook, and the decision to stay fit, you'll be on your way to eating like a champ.

George Foreman's Knock-Out-the-Fat Barbecue and Grilling Cookbook

NUTRIBITES

Look for Cherie's tidbits of nutrition information in this book. She's used her expertise as a nutritionist to create what she calls *nutribites*, nutrition tips that are given in "bites" throughout the cookbook. They make nutrition information as fun and accessible as possible. We hear a lot of negative information about what we should and shouldn't eat, which can get a bit depressing. As you leaf through the following pages, you may be pleasantly surprised to learn that some of your favorite foods contain more nutrients than you might expect. Powerful nutrients are found in surprising places. For example, would you have guessed that bell peppers have more than four times the vitamin C of oranges and orange juice? Or that garlic has natural antibiotic properties? Nutribites will also help you cut the fat in your diet by giving you healthful tips on what to choose when you shop for food. Nutribites can help you enjoy our recipes twice as much by knowing what they are contributing to your well-being.

COMMENTS ON THE NUTRITIONAL ANALYSES

To help monitor the amount of fat and other key nutrients you and your family consume, nutritional analyses are included for every recipe. All recipes with 30 percent or less total fat content, 10 percent or less saturated fat content, and 100 mg or less cholesterol content are indicated by this symbol: ♡

- In recipes that offer a range of servings (e.g., 4 to 6), the highest number (6) was picked.

- Optional ingredients have not been included in the analysis. For example, "salt to taste" is optional and was therefore excluded.

- Sometimes a recipe includes a suggestion to serve over rice, couscous, or pasta. The accompaniments are not included in the analysis.

- When a recipe analysis is based on a low-fat or low-sodium version of an ingredient, that is always specified in the recipe.

- When an option is given, the analysis is based on the leanest cut of meat, fish, or poultry.

- Skin was always removed for the poultry recipes. However, for analysis purposes, only the chicken breasts were analyzed with no skin.

CHAPTER TWO

GRILLING AND BARBECUING IN HEALTHFUL STYLE

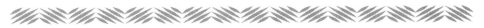

BARBECUING AND GRILLING HAVE BEEN POPULAR METHODS FOR roasting game for centuries. Native Americans built their own outdoor barbecues from green saplings and dried their meat and fish over a slowly smoldering fire. It is believed that colonists learned how to barbecue hogs from slaves, and that Native Americans used a vinegar-based sauce with their meat. French settlers roasted whole animals over open fires, calling it *barbe-a-queue.* Spaniards called the grilling process *barbacoa.*

Barbecuing or grilling was a regional phenomenon of the South and Midwest until after World War II, when suburban America embraced backyard grilling as part of the good life. Today, people spend nearly $500 million a year on barbecue sauce. An outdoor grill or barbecue is almost as important as a television set for the American family, and more grills than ever before are sizzling across America.

Almost every dish in *George Foreman's Knock-Out-the-Fat Barbecue and Grilling Cookbook* can be prepared on an outdoor grill or in an electric grilling machine in your kitchen. From the tender Ginger-Lime Swordfish (page 83) to the popular Rosemary-Thyme Chicken Strips over Lemon-Garlic Caesar Salad (page 130) to our Deluxe Turkey Burgers (page 55), there's a grilled or barbecued meal with fabulous flavor for almost any occasion.

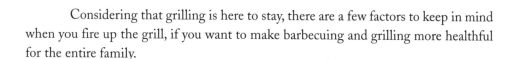
Considering that grilling is here to stay, there are a few factors to keep in mind when you fire up the grill, if you want to make barbecuing and grilling more healthful for the entire family.

Tips for Grilling Healthier Food

When wood or charcoal burns, chemicals known as benzopyrene and hetero-cyclic amines (HCAs) form that can cause genetic damage to cells, the first step in causing cancer. Benzopyrenes are formed in the smoke and flames from the barbecue, grill, or charcoal broiler. HCAs are formed when meat browns from the heat, a chemical reaction that transforms a protein in the meat muscle known as creatine into cell-damaging HCAs. Specifically, HCAs are linked to colon, breast, and pancreatic cancer. The higher and more prolonged the heat, the more the HCAs are embedded in the meat, poultry, or fish. Keeping this in mind, there are a number of things you can do to grill smarter and healthier.

1. Reduce carcinogenic chemicals by partially poaching or baking your food before placing it on the grill. (This does not apply to electric grilling machines.) Steaks eaten medium rare have the fewest unwanted chemicals. People who like their meat well done are at the most risk. (To kill *E. coli* bacteria and other harmful pathogens, cook burgers just until there is no pink and the juices run clear; do not char them.)

2. Add textured vegetable (soy) protein (TVP) to ground meat. It not only helps reduce the fat content but also blocks a large percentage of the HCAs. You can mix TVP with ground beef, pork, lamb, chicken, or turkey. The taste and texture won't change much (in fact, we think it improves), but the protective health benefits will greatly increase.

3. Scrape the black char off grilled meat, poultry, or fish, and remove charred skin. Black char contains cancer-promoting polycyclic aromatic carbons (PAHs) in addition to benzopyrene and HCAs.

4. Include garlic in your meal whenever you eat grilled or barbecued food. Studies show that certain chemicals in garlic block the destructive work of HCAs.

5. Use lean meat rather than fatty meat, which drips and causes more flames and smoke.

6. Cook food as far away from the coals as possible. You can also protect food by using foil or a pan to shield it from smoke and flames.

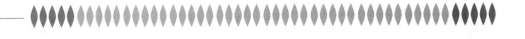

George Foreman's Knock-Out-the-Fat Barbecue and Grilling Cookbook

7. Cook food slowly at lower temperatures using the indirect method of barbecuing as often as possible. The temperature can be lowered by sprinkling water onto the coals or, in the case of a gas grill, by turning down the temperature regulator.

8. Use an electric grill or kitchen electric grilling machine; it produces no smoke and flames, and cooks food faster, thus reducing exposure time to high temperatures.

Fat-Reducing Tips

The American Heart Association, the American Dietetic Association, the U.S. Surgeon General, and the USDA all recommend that no more than 30 percent of our daily calorie intake come from fat. In addition to heart disease, studies show that eating too much animal fat is linked to certain types of cancer, including prostate and breast cancer. Here are some healthy ways to reduce the fat content in foods:

1. Cut sour cream and mayonnaise with equal amounts of nonfat or low-fat yogurt for a reduced-fat spread or topping.

2. For more flavor without adding extra fat, season foods with onion, garlic, spices, herbs, hot sauce, salsa, lemon juice, or vinegar.

3. Three to four ounces of meat, poultry, or fish is an ample serving for most adults, when combined with generous servings of plant-based foods. (Three ounces of meat is about the size of a deck of cards.) Children need only half this amount.

4. Choose the leanest cuts of meat, such as flank steak or round steak.

5. Trim all visible fat away from the meat.

6. Hamburger meat is very high in fat. Buy the leanest ground beef possible (about 90 percent lean). Ground, skinless chicken breast or skinless turkey breast is even lower in fat than 90 percent lean ground beef.

7. To reduce the saturated fat in a burger, cut back on the amount of meat and add plant-based ingredients such as TVP or oat bran to ground meat along with chopped vegetables. (Studies indicate that oat bran has cholesterol-lowering effects.)

8. When your taste buds demand a burger, grill your own. Avoid fast-food burgers. Some fast-food hamburgers and cheeseburgers contain 12 to 15 teaspoons of fat and tip the scales at over 700 calories.

9. Take the skin off chicken or turkey before cooking.

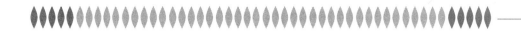

10. Eat onions and garlic with high-fat foods. A number of studies have indicated that onions eaten with a high-fat meal bring blood cholesterol down. Garlic has also demonstrated cholesterol-lowering abilities in numerous scientific studies.

Safety Tips for
Handling Meat, Poultry, and Fish

Every year many people become ill because of food mishandling at home. Hospital records indicate that food poisonings begin to rise in May and June and stay high until September, when they drop back to winter levels. We can protect ourselves against food-borne illnesses caused by parasites and bacterial pathogens like *Salmonella* and *E. coli* with some common-sense food preparation and serving practices in the kitchen and at outdoor cookouts and picnics. The following list of tips should help you stay healthier all year long.

Handling

1. Choose ground meat packages that are cold and tightly wrapped. The meat surface exposed to air should be red and the interior of fresh meat should be dark.

2. Place frozen and refrigerated foods in your cart near the end of your shopping, and make the grocery store your last stop, especially in warmer weather.

3. Place ground meat and ground poultry in the refrigerator or freezer as soon as you get home.

4. Defrost frozen meats in the refrigerator—not at room temperature.

Storage

1. Refrigerator temperatures should be set at 40°F or lower and the freezer at 0°F or colder.

2. Keep uncooked meat or poultry in the refrigerator and cook or freeze it within one to two days of purchase.

3. Use cooked meat or poultry stored in the refrigerator within three days.

Cleaning

1. Always wash your hands thoroughly with soap and hot water before preparing food and after handling raw meat, fish, or poultry.

Grilling and Barbecuing in Healthful Style

2. Don't allow raw meat, poultry, or fish juices to touch ready-to-eat foods either in the refrigerator or during food preparation.

3. Before transferring cooked food from the grill to the platter you used to carry it to the grill, be sure to wash the platter with hot, soapy water.

4. Wash the utensils that have touched the raw meat, poultry, or fish with hot, soapy water before using them for cooked foods.

5. *Salmonella* and other bacteria can live on work surfaces and get transferred easily to other foods you cut up. Wash the counters, cutting boards, or anything else that has come into contact with raw meats with hot, soapy water or place items in the dishwasher. Never use a wooden cutting board to cut up raw meat, poultry, or fish, since it is more difficult to clean all bacteria from the wood.

Cooking

1. Allow meat, fish, or poultry to sit at room temperature no more than 1 hour. Marinate foods in the refrigerator if more than 1 hour is desired.

2. Completely cook fish, poultry, and ground meat. Raw portions can carry bacteria and parasites and cause food-borne illnesses.

3. The center of ground meat and poultry patties should not be pink, and the juices should always run clear.

4. Ground meat patties are safe to eat when they reach 160°F in the center; ground poultry patties when their interior reaches 165°F.

5. When grilling meat, poultry, or fish, turn it over at least once to cook evenly.

6. Don't use leftover marinade from raw meat, poultry, or fish unless it's been thoroughly heated to kill all bacteria or parasites that might be present.

7. Refrigerate all leftovers within 2 hours after cooking or serving.

8. To reheat leftovers, cover and heat to 165°F, or until hot and steaming throughout.

For more safe handling and preparation information, contact the USDA's Meat and Poultry Hotline at (800) 535-4555.

FACTS ABOUT GRILLS AND GRILLING

THE TWO TYPES OF GRILLS ON WHICH WE TESTED OUR RECIPES are simple to use and inexpensive: a kettle-shaped charcoal grill and an electric grilling machine. Charcoal cooks foods at a lower heat, which is an advantage because the foods are less likely to burn and therefore should contain fewer fire-generated chemicals like benzopyrene, HCAs, and PAHs. (See page 21 for more information.) Also, the taste of charcoal-grilled foods is quite unbeatable. Charcoal grills take about 35 to 40 minutes to reach the right temperature for cooking, however, which is one reason gas grills have become popular.

Cherie and I also chose to prepare our recipes on an electric grilling machine because it is economical, can be used year-round, heats to the right cooking temperature in about 3 minutes, cooks nearly everything in under 5 minutes, is very easy to clean, and does not produce unhealthy, fire-induced chemicals.

With only a few exceptions, our recipes can be cooked on either charcoal, gas, or electric grills. The following information about the variety of grills on the market is designed to help you experience the best in grilling and barbecuing.

Purchasing a Grill and Accessories

You don't need a lot of special or expensive equipment to produce delicious, succulent meals. A basic grill and a few tools are all that's required.

Kettle-Shaped Grills

The kettle-shaped grill's unique design eliminates the need to control the heat by lowering and raising the grid. It minimizes flare-ups and produces quite even heat. Kettle-shaped grills are designed to be used with the lid closed. Vents in the lid and on the bottom provide adequate air flow to keep the fire going while preventing flare-ups. This type of grill allows the cook to sear the food without burning it. By moving the coals to the edges and inserting a drip pan in the center, food can be cooked slowly.

There are a couple of drawbacks to kettle-shaped grills. The lid is not hinged, which is an inconvenience at times, especially when frequent opening and closing are required. Also, the grid is not adjustable; you cannot move the food closer to the fire or farther away.

Rectangular Hinged Grills

The advantage of rectangular hinged charcoal grills is that you are able to raise or lower the grid. Also, a hinged lid makes opening and closing the lid easier. A drawback to this type of grill is that it is harder to clean out the ashes. And when it comes to even cooking, heat circulation, and preventing flare-ups, it's no match for the kettle-shaped grill.

Open Grills

Open grills include braziers, hibachis, and other lidless grills. A brazier is a charcoal grill that is a firebox and grid on a stand. (Be aware that the less expensive brands often have wobbly legs, which can be dangerous.) Open grills can be rectangular- or kettle-shaped with rounded undersides. They should have a charcoal rack that allows the air to flow around the fire and lets the ashes drop away from the burning coals. Hooded braziers offer a covering for half the surface. The drawback with open grills is that they are likely to experience flare-ups during cooking, since they don't have a lid. (Keep a spray bottle handy to control flare-ups.) They are best used for fish and lean meats, and when using fat-free marinades.

Gas Grills

Covered gas grills are the new generation of sophistication in outdoor cooking. Though more expensive than other types of grills, their ability to maintain even, medium heat with high-tech circulation and control has made them popular. You'll find either lava-rock or porcelain-coated metal versions. A fire grate near the burners holds the lava-rocks or ceramic bricks. They allow heat to emanate evenly from the gas burners and they vaporize drippings, thus giving the food a grilled flavor. The lava rocks are difficult to keep clean, however, and over time layers of burned grease can give food an unpleasant flavor. The porcelain-coated bricks, on the other hand, can be easily removed and are dishwasher safe.

One of the greatest advantages to cooking with a gas grill is the ability to control cooking temperatures. One of the drawbacks is the lack of a distinctive smoked flavor. And to some, cooking on a gas grill just doesn't have the lure of traditional charcoal-fire cooking.

Electric Grills

Electric grills create no fumes and are therefore suitable for indoor or outdoor use. Most do not have covers and come in tabletop models for the kitchen and larger models for the patio or deck. They have a metal box with an electric heating element near the bottom, with a bed of volcanic rocks touching the element. Because they do not produce smoke and flames, they will not create the unhealthy compounds in the meat that charcoal or gas grills produce. One drawback is that an electric outlet needs to be close enough for use. Another is the lack of the distinctive smoked flavor of outdoor grilling.

Indoor Electric Grilling Machines

Created for kitchen use, electric grilling machines are a fast, easy way to make grilled foods in a fraction of the time. They are small electric appliances that sear meat quickly and lock in juices. Most foods will cook in under 5 minutes. They are easy to clean, due to a nonstick surface. And they are healthful to use, since smoke and flames don't react with the meat to create unhealthy chemicals. One drawback is that the food lacks the distinctive smoked flavor of outdoor grilling. Also, some foods don't cook well because of large bones or because of their size. Thick ribs or big pork chops take so long to cook that the outer portion gets dry and tough before the interior is done.

Accessories

Basting Brush

For many of our recipes a basting brush is essential, but you don't need to spend a lot of money for a fancy brush. A simple twisted-wire-handled brush works just fine for grilling outdoors. A long-handled, larger brush is nice for oiling the grid.

Drip Pan

A drip pan is best for barbecuing so the food can cook over indirect heat. We recommend 2- to 3-inch-deep disposable rectangular aluminum pans you can throw away after use.

Griffo Grill

This is a special rack with small holes for grilling small portions of food or those with coatings, like George's Catfish Fillets with Sesame Crust (page 92). This rack can be purchased at most stores that specialize in grills and grilling accessories.

Grill Brush and Scraper

Though a heavy-duty scrubbing pad will work, a grill brush is your best bet to keep the grid clean. This inexpensive accessory is very handy for removing any food particles or burned-on grease after cooking, while the grid is still warm. Following this procedure, you shouldn't have to wash the grid with soap and water, which removes the seasoning from it.

Heavy Aluminum Foil

We use heavy-duty aluminum foil to make little tents for grilled vegetables and to place under some foods while they are cooking.

Hinged Wire Baskets

These are two grills secured by a latch that hold fish, hamburger, sausage patties, or bread. Simply oil the basket, put the food inside, and place the basket over the heat. Flip the basket when one side is done.

Insulated Oven Mitts

Regular kitchen pot holders won't protect you from the heat as you turn food or lift the lid of the grill. Long, insulated oven mitts are a good idea for outdoor grilling.

Long-Handled Metal Utensils

Long-handled spatulas, forks, and tongs are very helpful for turning food.

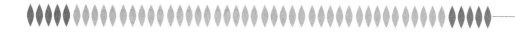

Plastic Cover for the Grill

Unless your grill is stored indoors, a plastic cover is essential to protect it.

Skewers

Either metal or bamboo skewers can be used for kabobs. Metal skewers never catch on fire, but they also need to be washed. Bamboo skewers, which we recommend in our recipes, need to be soaked in water for 15 to 30 minutes before using to prevent their burning.

Spray Bottle

Though there aren't many flare-ups with kettle or gas grills, it's always a good idea to have a spray bottle filled with water nearby in case of an emergency.

Lighting the Fire

Ever feel confused when you look at all the different briquettes and wood charcoals? A wide variety of products have entered the market, which can leave you wondering where to start. The traditional charcoal briquettes are now surrounded by "instant lighting" briquettes, hardwood charcoal, hardwood-flavored charcoal, and smoke-creating hardwood chips, chunks, and sawdust. Each is appropriate for different situations, and you can judge which one is right for your needs.

Charcoal Briquettes

Because they burn evenly and consistently, charcoal briquettes are still the fuel of choice for about half of today's consumers. Most briquettes are made from scrap wood, bound with fillers and additives, and pressed into shape. Instant-lighting briquettes are made by adding petroleum products. Wait until the briquettes are covered with a thin layer of gray ash (about 20 to 30 minutes after lighting) before placing your food on the grill. This will allow the additives to burn off. Use 30 to 40 briquettes, which will allow about 1 hour of cooking time. If you are cooking a food very slowly and the heat dies out, be aware that adding new briquettes will also create new fumes from the additives burning off. You could start your coals in another place, like a metal can, and then add them to the grill when a layer of ash has formed on them.

Hardwood Charcoals

Mesquite charcoal is by far the most popular, most economical, and most available of the hardwoods. Mesquite charcoal (and all other hardwoods) is carbonized by slow smoldering. It burns much hotter than charcoal briquettes and imbues a subtle, smoky flavor to food. Leftover pieces can be reused. One distinct advantage is that it (and all other hardwood charcoals) have no added fillers or additives. One caution, however: It tends to pop burning embers into the air and needs to be constantly supervised. Other hardwood charcoals, such as apple, cherry, hickory, maple, and oak, impart a flavorful, smoky taste. Several drawbacks are their price, scarcity, and inability to burn as hot as mesquite. Two or three pounds of any hardwood charcoal should be sufficient for an hour of cooking.

Hardwood Chips, Chunks, and Sawdust

To add distinctive flavor to foods, you can use chunks, chips, or sawdust from any hardwood, such as ash, apple, cherry, grapevine, hickory, maple, or oak. Avoid pine and other softwoods as their resins produce an unpleasant aftertaste. Hardwood chips work best for a gas grill and should be soaked in water for 30 minutes before using. Place the water-soaked chips in an old pan toward the back corner of the grill. Sawdust works very well also for gas grills. Place sawdust in an old pan on top of lava rocks or bars. Turn the burner to high underneath the pan just until the sawdust starts to smolder and then turn it off.

Fire Starters

Kindling

Several sheets of newspaper can be crumpled or twisted into rolls and placed on the bottom of the grill. On top place a handful of dry kindling, and a half-dozen briquettes on top of that. Light the newspaper and, hopefully, the briquettes should catch on fire. If they do not, add more newspaper and kindling. Once the briquettes light, add the desired number of briquettes (about thirty) until you achieve the right fire.

Lighter Fluids and Jellied Fire Lighters

To use a commercial lighter fluid, carefully pour or spray the fluid onto a pyramid of charcoal. Allow the fluid to permeate the charcoal before igniting it with a long match. Never squirt the fluid onto a burning fire. Flames can travel back up the stream and set your hands or arms, or the entire can of fluid, on fire. Be careful that excess fluid does not collect in the bottom of the grill. Never use gasoline, naphtha, paint thinner, or kerosene, as they are too flammable. Only buy products that are labeled for use in grills and barbecues.

If you choose a jellied fire lighter, put several teaspoons of jelly between the charcoals in the base of the charcoal pyramid. Wait several minutes and ignite.

Electric Starters

To use an electric starter, place the loop of the heating element near the base of the charcoal pyramid. In about 10 minutes, the fire should be started. Remove your starter right after the fire starts or the heating element will be damaged. The one drawback to this type of fire starter is that you need to be near an electrical outlet.

Outdoor Cooking Methods

Grilling

Foods that are cooked directly over a heat source, seared to seal in the juices, and have the distinctive grill marks are considered grilled foods. Grilling lends itself especially well to foods that are low in fat, such as fish and poultry, and others that don't take very long to cook, such as hamburgers, vegetables, kabobs, and thin cuts of meat. If using a kettle-shaped grill, always keep the lid closed, except when basting or turning the food. If you are using a gas grill, turn all three burners to high and close the lid. In about 10 minutes the grill should be hot enough. You can leave the burners on high or turn one or two burners down, depending on the food being cooked and the desired result.

Barbecuing

To barbecue means to cook food over a cool, smoky fire. Most barbecued food is basted with a tangy sauce at the end and served with the same sauce at the table. Grilled food is cooked more quickly than barbecued food. You can barbecue spareribs, country-style ribs, beef ribs, beef short ribs, chicken, or fish. To barbecue in a kettle-shaped grill, prepare the coals as you would for grilling. When they are covered with a light ash, separate them into two piles on each side of the grill. Place a drip pan (disposable aluminum pans are the easiest) in the middle. Add presoaked hardwood chips or chunks to the charcoal piles at this time, if using. Allow the grill to heat for about 5

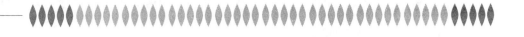

minutes. Sear the food for about 3 minutes on each side directly over the heat source, and then move it directly over the drip pan and close the lid. If you are using a gas grill, prepare it as you would for grilling. After 10 minutes, turn off the center burner and place the drip pan over it. Place your food directly over the drip pan and close the lid.

Cooking Times

Though approximate cooking times are provided with every recipe, they are general recommendations. The time in which the food is done may be quite different from what is noted in the recipe, because grills vary, climate influences temperature, and altitude has an effect on how long it takes something to cook. It is important to watch your food closely so that it is neither undercooked nor overcooked. Use the cooking times in the recipes as ballpark ranges.

C H A P T E R F O U R

MARINADES

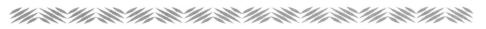

MARINADES ARE WINNING CONTRIBUTIONS TO GRILLING BECAUSE
they add so much flavor, prevent drying, and tenderize poultry, meat, and fish. You can
marinate foods for at least an hour, overnight, or even longer, depending on the inten-
sity of flavor desired. Foods that marinate for 1 hour can be left at room temperature;
otherwise, marinating should be done in the refrigerator. Before grilling, allow refrigerated food to warm to room temperature (approximately 30 minutes).

Zesty Fat-Free Marinade ♡

A great marinade for fish or chicken, this oil-free combination lends bursts of flavor, especially to mild-flavored fish.

Juice of ½ lemon
1 garlic clove, finely chopped
2 tablespoons white wine
1 tablespoon lemon zest

2 teaspoons tarragon vinegar
1 teaspoon dried tarragon
¼ teaspoon freshly ground black pepper

In a medium bowl, combine all the ingredients, mixing well, and set aside until ready to use.

Preparation time: *5 minutes*
Makes about ½ cup

Nutritional Breakdown (1 tablespoon per serving)

Calories: 5	*Carbohydrates: 1 gm*	*Cholesterol: 0 mg*	*Saturated fat: 0 gm*
Protein: 0 gm	*Sodium: 0 mg*	*Fat: 0 gm*	*% calories fat: 0*

Fat-Free Garlic-Wine Marinade ♡

This flavorful marinade, which uses no oil, is appropriate for chicken or beef. The balsamic vinegar makes it too assertive for fish.

¼ cup balsamic vinegar
¼ cup sweet Marsala, sherry, or sweet
    white wine
2 tablespoons fresh lemon juice
2 tablespoons chopped fresh oregano or
    1 tablespoon dried

2 tablespoons chopped fresh basil or
    1 tablespoon dried
¼ teaspoon freshly ground black pepper
4 garlic cloves, minced

In a medium bowl, combine all the ingredients, mixing well, and set aside until ready to use.

Preparation time: *5 minutes*
Makes about ¾ cup

Nutritional Breakdown (1 tablespoon per serving)

Calories: 13	*Carbohydrates: 2 gm*	*Cholesterol: 0 mg*	*Saturated fat: 0 gm*
Protein: 0 gm	*Sodium: 0 mg*	*Fat: 0 gm*	*% calories fat: 0*

Rosemary-Thyme Marinade

This tangy, herbed marinade is good for chicken and fish.

½ cup extra-virgin olive oil
¼ cup fresh lemon juice
2 garlic cloves, pressed

1 teaspoon dried thyme
1 teaspoon dried rosemary
½ teaspoon lemon zest

In a small bowl, combine all the ingredients, mixing well, and set aside until ready to use.

Preparation time: *5 minutes*
Makes about ¾ cup

Nutritional Breakdown (1 tablespoon per serving)

Calories: 82	*Carbohydrates: 1 gm*	*Cholesterol: 0 mg*	*Saturated fat: 1 gm*
Protein: 0 gm	*Sodium: 0 mg*	*Fat: 9 gm*	*% calories fat: 96%*

Raspberry Vinegar Marinade

This light, tangy, sweet marinade complements vegetable kabobs, fish, or chicken.

¼ cup extra-virgin olive oil
¼ cup raspberry vinegar
¼ cup chopped green onions
1 tablespoon fresh lemon juice

1 tablespoon honey
1 tablespoon minced garlic
2 teaspoons dried thyme
¼ teaspoon freshly ground black pepper

In a medium bowl, combine all the ingredients, mixing well, and set aside until ready to use.

Preparation time: *5 minutes*
Makes about 1 cup

Nutritional Breakdown (1 tablespoon per serving)

Calories: 35	*Carbohydrates: 2 gm*	*Cholesterol: 0 mg*	*Saturated fat: 0 gm*
Protein: 0 gm	*Sodium: 0 mg*	*Fat: 3 gm*	*% calories fat: 83%*

Ginger-Soy Marinade

Spicy and with an Asian influence, this marinade goes well with beef or chicken.

¼ cup chopped green onions   *2 tablespoons honey*
¼ cup toasted sesame oil   *2 tablespoons minced garlic*
¼ cup light soy sauce or tamari   *1 tablespoon minced ginger*
¼ cup Marsala or Madeira wine

In a medium bowl, combine all the ingredients and set aside until ready to use.

Preparation time: *5 minutes*
Makes about 1¼ cups

Nutritional Breakdown (1 tablespoon per serving)

Calories: 33	*Carbohydrates: 2 gm*	*Cholesterol: 0 mg*	*Saturated fat: 0 gm*
Protein: 0 gm	*Sodium: 175 mg*	*Fat: 3 gm*	*% calories fat: 69%*

DRY RUBS

Dry rubs, or "dry" marinades, are blends of herbs and spices. They can be dry or they can be mixed with a small amount of liquid such as oil or alcohol. They add intense flavor to foods. Rinse and dry the fish, poultry, or meat and lightly oil the surface, if no liquid is used in the rub. Use about 1 to 2 tablespoons of the mixture per pound of food and spread over the flesh. Gently rub or press the mixture in to make sure it sticks. Let the food stand at room temperature for 30 minutes to an hour before grilling. If you wish to marinate longer, be sure to do so in the refrigerator.

Thyme–Bay Leaf Rub ♡

A nice herb blend for fish, especially fatty fish like halibut, sturgeon, or whitefish.

2 bay leaves
2 tablespoons dried thyme

2 teaspoons black peppercorns

Place all the ingredients in a spice grinder or food processor, and crush until well blended. Lightly oil the fish or chicken, and with your fingers press the herb blend into the flesh.

Preparation time: *about 3 minutes*
Makes about 2½ tablespoons

Nutritional Breakdown (1 teaspoon per serving)

Calories: 4	*Carbohydrates: 1 gm*	*Cholesterol: 0 mg*	*Saturated fat: 0 gm*
Protein: 0 gm	*Sodium: 0 mg*	*Fat: 0 gm*	*% calories fat: 0*

Cajun Spice Rub for Fish ♡

Substitute this dry rub for the marinade and sesame seeds used in George's Catfish Fillets with Sesame Crust (page 92) to grill a Cajun-style blackened catfish.

1 tablespoon paprika
2 teaspoons dried lemon zest
2 teaspoons coarsely ground black pepper
1 teaspoon dried tarragon

1 teaspoon dried basil
½ teaspoon cayenne pepper
¼ teaspoon salt

Mix all the ingredients together in a small bowl. Brush the fish lightly with canola oil, sprinkle about ½ teaspoon of dry rub over each side of the fish, and press it in with your fingers. Let the fish marinate at room temperature for 30 minutes to an hour before grilling.

Preparation time: *2 minutes*
Makes about 3 tablespoons

Nutritional Breakdown (1 teaspoon per serving)

Calories: 5	*Carbohydrates: 1 gm*	*Cholesterol: 0 mg*	*Saturated fat: 0 gm*
Protein: 0 gm	*Sodium: 65 mg*	*Fat: 0 gm*	*% calories fat: 0*

Garlic-Herb Rub

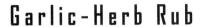 This herb blend goes well with lamb or beef. An alcohol base such as cognac or brandy can be substituted for the olive oil.

1 tablespoon extra-virgin olive oil   *½ teaspoon dried oregano*
1 teaspoon finely minced garlic   *½ teaspoon dried basil*
1 teaspoon crushed sage   *Pinch cayenne pepper*

Mix all the ingredients together in a small bowl. Use ½ teaspoon of the rub for each side of the meat and rub the mixture into the meat. Let the meat marinate for 30 minutes to an hour at room temperature before grilling.

Preparation time: *5 minutes*
Makes about 2 tablespoons

Nutritional Breakdown (1 teaspoon per serving)

Calories: 21	*Carbohydrates: 0 gm*	*Cholesterol: 0 mg*	*Saturated fat: 0 gm*
Protein: 0 gm	*Sodium: 0 mg*	*Fat: 2 gm*	*% calories fat: 94%*

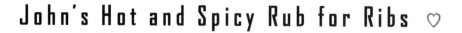

John's Hot and Spicy Rub for Ribs ♡

Sprinkle this spicy blend over beef or pork ribs and rub it in. Barbecue the ribs over indirect heat, being careful not to overcook them. Finish with your favorite sauce, like the Louisiana Bacon Barbecue Sauce (page 145) or South Carolina Mustard Sauce (page 44). We're sure someone will say these are the best ribs they've ever tasted!

1 tablespoon freshly ground black pepper	$\frac{1}{2}$ teaspoon ground red pepper
1 tablespoon paprika	$\frac{1}{4}$ teaspoon dry mustard
$\frac{1}{2}$ tablespoon chili powder	$\frac{1}{8}$ teaspoon ground cinnamon
$\frac{1}{2}$ teaspoon celery salt	

Mix all the ingredients together in a small bowl. Brush the meat with a little canola oil, sprinkle the dry rub over the ribs, and press it in with a spoon or your fingers. Let the meat marinate for 30 minutes to an hour at room temperature.

Preparation time: *5 minutes*
Makes about 3 tablespoons

Nutritional Breakdown (1 teaspoon per serving)

Calories: 6	Carbohydrates: 1 gm	Cholesterol: 0 mg	Saturated fat: 0 gm
Protein: 0 gm	Sodium: 118 mg	Fat: 0 gm	% calories fat: 0

Spice and Herb Rub for Lamb ♡

This blend makes the Spice-and-Herb-Crusted Lamb with Yogurt Sauce (page 108) extra delicious.

1 tablespoon paprika
2 teaspoons coarsely ground black pepper
2 teaspoons dried rosemary
1 teaspoon crushed fennel seed (crushed with a mortar and pestle)

1 teaspoon dried oregano
1 teaspoon dried basil
½ teaspoon dried thyme
½ teaspoon cayenne pepper
¼ teaspoon salt (optional)

Preparation time: *5 minutes*
Makes about 4 tablespoons

Nutritional Breakdown (1 teaspoon per serving)

Calories: 5
Protein: 0 gm
Carbohydrates: 1 gm
Sodium: 0 mg
Cholesterol: 0 mg
Fat: 0 gm
Saturated fat: 0 gm
% calories fat: 0

C H A P T E R   S I X

BARBECUE SAUCES

JUST FOR FUN, CHERIE AND I THOUGHT YOU MIGHT ENJOY KNOW-
ing that the word *barbecue* was once street slang for a good-looking woman, and it's the
reason why Louis Armstrong's 1927 song was called "Struttin' with Some Barbecue."
Today, barbecue means only one thing: finger-lickin' good meat, poultry, or fish cooked
slowly over a fire. Most barbecue is served with a tangy sauce to flavor and moisten the
meat. There are many regional versions of the sauce that carry the town or state name
where they originated, like Kansas City, Carolina, or Texas barbecue sauce. We've
adapted several regional recipes, adding a few of our own favorite ingredients.

LBJ's Texas Barbecue Sauce ♡

If you've read my autobiography, *By George,* then you know how much Lyndon B.
Johnson's Job Corps meant to me. It gave me a second chance to complete high school
and gain valuable job skills, and it's where I started boxing. In honor of the first president to host a barbecue at the White House, Cherie and I have adapted LBJ's sweet,
mild barbecue sauce, which is excellent for beef or pork ribs.

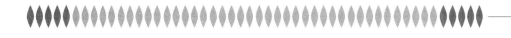

1–2 tablespoons extra-virgin olive oil
½ large onion, finely chopped
½ green bell pepper, finely chopped
2–3 garlic cloves, minced
1 cup tomato puree
½ cup apple cider vinegar

½ cup chili sauce
3 tablespoons honey
2 tablespoons Worcestershire sauce
6 peppercorns or ½ teaspoon coarsely ground
    black pepper
1 bay leaf

1. Heat the oil in a medium pan over medium-high heat, and add the onion, bell pepper, and garlic. Cook for about 10 minutes, or until tender.
2. Add all the remaining ingredients, mixing well, and bring to a boil. Reduce the heat to low and simmer for 1 hour.
3. Strain or serve chunky, whichever you prefer, as a finishing and table sauce. (LBJ's was strained.)

Preparation time: *about 10 minutes*
Cooking time: *1 hour and 10 minutes*
Makes about 2 cups

Nutritional Breakdown (2 tablespoons per serving)

Calories: 44	Carbohydrates: 9 gm	Cholesterol: 0 mg	Saturated fat: 0 gm
Protein: 1 gm	Sodium: 183 mg	Fat: 1 gm	% calories fat: 16%

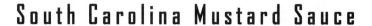

South Carolina Mustard Sauce

South Carolina's regional sauces have a variety of bases. The area around Columbia is known for its mustard base. Tart and tangy, this recipe is great on pork or chicken. With this sauce and John's Hot and Spicy Rub for Ribs (page 40), you'll barbecue some of the best country-style ribs you've ever eaten.

¾ cup yellow mustard
¾ cup red wine vinegar
¼ cup honey
1 tablespoon canola oil
2 teaspoons Worcestershire sauce

1 teaspoon butter
1 teaspoon freshly ground black pepper
½ teaspoon salt
½ teaspoon hot sauce

1. In a medium saucepan, combine all the ingredients and mix well.
2. Simmer over low heat for about 30 minutes. Let sit at room temperature for 1 hour before using.
3. Unused sauce can be refrigerated for several weeks or frozen. (Add 2 to 4 tablespoons of water to reconstitute.)

Preparation time: *5 minutes*
Cooking time: *about 30 minutes*
Makes about 2 cups

Nutritional Breakdown (2 tablespoons per serving)

Calories: 50	*Carbohydrates: 8 gm*	*Cholesterol: 0 mg*	*Saturated fat: 0 gm*
Protein: 1 gm	*Sodium: 204 mg*	*Fat: 2 gm*	*% calories fat: 36%*

Sweet Vinegar Barbecue Sauce

America's original barbecue sauce was vinegar-based. It was Native Americans and slaves who taught the colonists how to barbecue hogs. To enhance flavor and cover up bad meat, they used a tomatoless vinegar baste that was derived from the English "ketchup" of the time. This Sweet Vinegar Barbecue Sauce goes especially well with chicken or fish.

¹⁄₄ cup red wine vinegar
¹⁄₄ cup extra-virgin olive oil
¹⁄₄ cup honey
2 tablespoons dried basil
1 tablespoon dried oregano

¹⁄₄ teaspoon freshly ground black pepper
Juice of ¹⁄₂ lemon
2 garlic cloves, minced
1 teaspoon grated lemon zest
1 green onion, chopped

1. Add the vinegar, olive oil, honey, basil, oregano, pepper, lemon juice, and garlic to a medium saucepan, and bring to a boil over medium-high heat. Turn the heat to low and cook for about 15 minutes, or until the sauce is reduced by about one half. Remove from the heat and stir in the lemon zest and green onion.
2. Serve warm as a finishing and table sauce.
3. Unused sauce will keep for several weeks in the refrigerator.

Preparation time: *5 minutes*
Cooking time: *about 18 minutes*
Makes about ¹⁄₂ cup

Nutritional Breakdown (per serving)

Calories: 197	*Carbohydrates: 20 gm*	*Cholesterol: 0 mg*	*Saturated fat: 2 gm*
Protein: 0 gm	*Sodium: 0 mg*	*Fat: 14 gm*	*% calories fat: 60%*

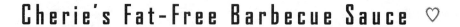

Cherie's Fat-Free Barbecue Sauce ♡

You don't have to add fat to create great flavor. This fat-free sauce is delicious with beef or chicken.

1 (10 ¾ ounce) can tomato puree
¼ cup honey
¼ cup blackstrap molasses
2 tablespoons light soy sauce or tamari
1 tablespoon balsamic vinegar

½ teaspoon ground cinnamon
½ teaspoon ground allspice
¼ teaspoon freshly ground black pepper
⅛ teaspoon cayenne pepper
2 garlic cloves, pressed

In a medium saucepan, combine all the ingredients and simmer on low heat for about 30 minutes, or until the sauce thickens.

Preparation: about 5 minutes
Cooking time: about 30 minutes
Makes about 2 cups

Nutritional Breakdown (2 tablespoons per serving)

Calories: 74	Carbohydrates: 20 gm	Cholesterol: 0 mg	Saturated fat: 0 gm
Protein: 1 gm	Sodium: 318 mg	Fat: 0 gm	% calories fat: 0

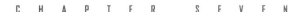

BURGERS
AND SANDWICHES

WITHOUT SOME PLANNING, A BURGER WITH ALL THE TRIMMINGS, like a thick slice of cheese, a layer of bacon, and a slathering of mayonnaise, can pack in over 40 grams of fat and reach over 700 calories. You can keep your burgers on the lighter side by choosing the leanest meat, whole-wheat buns, reduced-fat cheese, and reduced-fat mayonnaise or, instead of mayo, mustard.

If you're careful about the size of the meat patties, you can save even more fat and calories. Shape the meat into 4-ounce patties; when cooked, they'll result in satisfying 3-ounce burgers. Better yet, substitute chopped vegetables and bread crumbs, textured vegetable (soy) protein (TVP), or oat bran for some of the meat, and you'll lower the fat and calories even more, as Cherie and I did in George's Powerburger (page 48).

Choosing ground, skinless turkey or chicken to make your burgers lets you lower the fat content further. Add chopped vegetables and bread crumbs, TVP, or oat bran to the ground poultry meat as well, as we've done with the Grilled Santa Fe Chicken Burgers (page 54) and the Deluxe Turkey Burgers (page 55). Try a vegetarian burger for a truly healthful change (page 61) and see if your family even notices. We think ours are so good that even if they do, no one will care.

One thing is very important to remember: Always wash the platter you used to carry raw meat to your grill before serving any food on it.

George's Powerburger

〰 Healthier than its all-meat cousin, this hamburger boasts less fat and more flavor with the addition of plant-based ingredients, which replace some of the meat. The burger goes well with a green salad or potato salad. (This recipe is adapted from Cherie's book *The Healthy Gourmet,* published by Clarkson Potter.)

¼ cup chopped vegetables, such as yellow onions, green onions, zucchini, yellow squash, or red bell pepper
1 teaspoon canola oil, plus extra for the grid if using a grill
1 teaspoon water

¾ pound lean ground beef (90 percent lean contains the least fat)
¼ cup plain or seasoned bread crumbs or TVP (textured vegetable [soy] protein)
2 tablespoons chopped fresh parsley
4 buns (preferably whole wheat), lightly toasted

1. In a small skillet, sauté the vegetables in oil and water over medium-high heat until tender yet crisp, 8 to 10 minutes.
2. In a medium bowl, combine the vegetables, ground beef, bread crumbs or TVP, and parsley, and mix until well combined. With lightly moistened hands, form the mixture into four 4-inch patties.
3. Prepare the grill or electric grilling machine for cooking.
4. If using a charcoal grill, place the patties on the hottest area of a lightly oiled grid over ashen coals for 1 to 2 minutes on each side to brown. Move the patties to a cooler part of the grill and continue to cook for another 3 to 4 minutes on each side, or until the meat is thoroughly cooked (no pink remains and the juices run clear) and the patties spring back to the touch. When the burgers are nearly done, toast the buns on the coolest part of the grill.
5. If using an electric grilling machine, grill the patties for about 4 minutes, or until the meat is thoroughly cooked (no pink remains and the juices run clear) and the patties spring back to the touch. While the burgers are cooking, toast the buns in a skillet lightly brushed with oil or grill them in the machine for about 1 minute when the meat is done.
6. Place a meat patty on each bun and add your favorite condiments and toppings, such as dark leafy green lettuce or spinach, onion, and thinly sliced tomatoes.

Preparation time: *10 minutes*
Cooking time: *8–12 minutes on a grill; about 4 minutes in an electric grilling machine*
Makes 4 servings

Nutritional Breakdown (per serving)

Calories: 495	*Carbohydrates: 55 gm*	*Cholesterol: 53 mg*	*Saturated fat: 4 gm*
Protein: 25 gm	*Sodium: 169 mg*	*Fat: 19 gm*	*% calories fat: 35%*

Nutribite ≋

For the most nutritious burgers, place your meat patties on whole-wheat buns. Along with their higher content of fiber, B vitamins, vitamin E, magnesium, and other minerals, whole-wheat buns contain 1 less fat gram than regular or reduced-calorie buns. And when it comes to condiments, mustard is a good choice, sporting only 1 gram of fat. Top your burgers in healthful style with dark green leafy lettuce, fresh cilantro, basil, or spinach, and add a big bite of beta-carotene to boot.

Green Chili and Red Pepper Burgers with Roasted Red Pepper Mayonnaise

≋ The zip of green chilis and piquancy of roasted red peppers make this burger a delicious change from the norm.

³⁄₄ pound lean ground beef (90 percent lean contains the least fat)
¹⁄₄ cup unseasoned bread crumbs
1–2 tablespoons diced green chilies
¹⁄₂ teaspoon salt (optional)

Canola oil for the grid, if using a grill
1 red bell pepper, roasted, peeled, seeded, and sliced in strips (see note, page 50)
4 hamburger buns (preferably whole wheat), lightly toasted

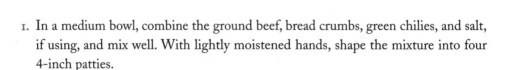

1. In a medium bowl, combine the ground beef, bread crumbs, green chilies, and salt, if using, and mix well. With lightly moistened hands, shape the mixture into four 4-inch patties.

2. Prepare the grill or electric grilling machine for cooking.

3. If using a charcoal grill, place the patties over ashen coals on the hottest area of a lightly oiled grill for 1 to 2 minutes on each side to brown. Then move the patties to the outside of the grid and continue to cook for another 3 to 4 minutes on each side, or until the meat is thoroughly cooked (no pink remains and the juices run clear) and the patties spring back to the touch. When the burgers are nearly done, toast the buns on the coolest part of the grill.

4. If using an electric grilling machine, grill the patties for 4 minutes, or until the meat is thoroughly cooked (no pink remains and the juices run clear) and the patties spring back to the touch. While the burgers are cooking, toast the buns in a skillet lightly brushed with oil or on the grilling machine when the meat is done.

5. Cut the roasted red bell pepper in strips. Spread the buns with Roasted Red Pepper Mayonnaise (page 51), add the meat patties and 2 or 3 strips of roasted red pepper and any other toppings you like, such as lettuce or sliced onions.

Preparation time: *10 minutes*
Cooking time: *8–12 minutes on a grill; about 4 minutes in an electric griller*
Makes 4 servings

Nutritional Breakdown (per serving without Roasted Red Pepper Mayonnaise)

Calories: 487	*Carbohydrates: 55 gm*	*Cholesterol: 52 mg*	*Saturated fat: 4 gm*
Protein: 25 gm	*Sodium: 18 mg*	*Fat: 18 gm*	*% calories fat: 33%*

See page 160 for roasting peppers on the grill. To roast in the oven, turn the oven to broil. Prick the peppers with a fork and place them in a shallow baking dish. Broil until the skins turn black, turning the peppers so the skin blackens all around, about 10 minutes. Don't worry if you hear them popping; that's normal. Place the peppers in a plastic or brown paper bag to cool (the steam will help loosen the skins), then peel and discard the seeds, ribs, and stems.

Roasted Red Pepper Mayonnaise

A nutritional bonus is the red peppers, which boast a generous helping of vitamin C—over four times that found in orange juice.

1 egg plus 1 yolk, at room temperature
2 tablespoons fresh lemon juice
2 teaspoons Dijon mustard
Salt and pepper to taste (optional)

1 cup canola oil
2 red bell peppers, roasted, peeled, and
    seeded, about 1 cup

1. In the bowl of a blender or food processor fitted with a steel blade, add the eggs, lemon juice, mustard, and salt and pepper, if desired, and process for 10 seconds.
2. With the motor running, slowly add the oil drop by drop, and then gradually increase the amount as the mixture thickens.
3. Add the red bell peppers and blend until the mixture is creamy.
4. Adjust the seasoning.
5. Refrigerate for at least 2 hours before serving; the mixture will thicken in the refrigerator.

Preparation time: *15 minutes*
Makes approximately 2 cups

Nutritional Breakdown (1 teaspoon per serving)

Calories: 22	*Carbohydrates: 0 gm*	*Cholesterol: 4 mg*	*Saturated fat: 0 gm*
Protein: 0 gm	*Sodium: 3 mg*	*Fat: 2 gm*	*% calories fat: 95%*

Chicken Burgers
with Onion-Dill Sauce ♡

Flavorful and tender describe these reduced-fat chicken burgers. We bet your family and guests will never guess they aren't eating beef unless you tell them. Try the Onion-Dill Sauce in place of mayonnaise for less fat with great flavor.

³⁄₄ pound ground, skinless chicken breast
¹⁄₄ cup unseasoned bread crumbs or TVP
    (textured vegetable [soy] protein)
2 tablespoons chopped fresh dill, or
    1¹⁄₂ teaspoons dried
¹⁄₂ teaspoon fresh thyme, or ¹⁄₄ teaspoon dried

¹⁄₂ teaspoon salt (optional)
¹⁄₄ teaspoon freshly ground black pepper
Canola oil for the grid, if using a grill
4 hamburger buns (preferably whole
    wheat), lightly toasted

1. In a medium bowl, combine the ground chicken, bread crumbs or TVP, dill, thyme, salt, if using, and pepper, and mix well. With lightly moistened hands, form the mixture into four 4-inch patties.
2. Prepare the grill or electric grilling machine for cooking.
3. If using a charcoal grill, place the patties on the hottest area of a lightly oiled grid over ashen coals for 1 to 2 minutes on each side to brown. Move the patties to the coolest part of the grill and continue to cook for another 3 to 4 minutes on each side, or until the meat is cooked thoroughly (no pink remains and the juices run clear) and the patties spring back to the touch. When the burgers are nearly done, toast the buns on the coolest part of the grill.
4. If using an electric grilling machine, grill the patties for about 4 minutes, or until the meat is cooked thoroughly (no pink remains and the juices run clear) and the patties spring back to the touch. While the burgers are cooking, toast the buns in a skillet lightly brushed with oil or toast for about 1 minute in the grilling machine when the meat is done.
5. Spread the buns with Onion-Dill Sauce and serve immediately.

Preparation time: *10 minutes*
Cooking time: *8–12 minutes on a grill; about 4 minutes in an electric griller*
Makes 4 servings

Nutritional Breakdown (per serving without the Onion-Dill Sauce)

Calories: 423	*Carbohydrates: 54 gm*	*Cholesterol: 52 mg*	*Saturated fat: 1 gm*
Protein: 27 gm	*Sodium: 169 mg*	*Fat: 10 gm*	*% calories fat: 21%*

Onion-Dill Sauce

2 tablespoons reduced-fat mayonnaise   *1 tablespoon finely chopped dill pickle*
2 tablespoons plain low-fat yogurt   *1 tablespoon fresh dill, or 1½ teaspoons dried*
1 tablespoon finely chopped onion

In a small bowl, combine all the ingredients, cover, and refrigerate until ready to serve.

Preparation time: *5 minutes*
Makes about ½ cup

Nutritional Breakdown (1 tablespoon per serving)

Calories: 13	*Carbohydrates: 1 gm*	*Cholesterol: 0 mg*	*Saturated fat: 0 gm*
Protein: 0 gm	*Sodium: 54 mg*	*Fat: 1 gm*	*% calories fat: 73%*

Nutribite 〰

Chicken is a healthy substitute for ground beef. Compared to 90 percent lean ground beef, 4 ounces of chicken has less fat, with only 2 grams of fat versus 9 grams. In addition, chicken contains 50 fewer calories than the leanest ground beef. These numbers, however, are based on ground chicken breast with no skin. You may need to ask your butcher to grind boneless, skinless chicken breast or grind it yourself at home.

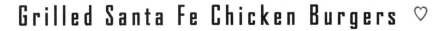

Grilled Santa Fe Chicken Burgers ♡

If you have a yen for Southwestern food, you should enjoy these Santa Fe–inspired burgers. Roasted Red Pepper Mayonnaise (page 51) goes well with these burgers, too. They're good with a green salad or a cup of chilled gazpacho.

³⁄₄ pound ground, skinless chicken breast
¹⁄₄ cup unseasoned bread crumbs or TVP
(textured vegetable [soy] protein)
¹⁄₄ cup finely chopped red bell pepper
¹⁄₄ cup chopped green onions
1–2 tablespoons diced green chilies

¹⁄₂ teaspoon salt (optional)
¹⁄₄ teaspoon ground black pepper
Canola oil for the grid, if using a grill
4 hamburger buns (preferably whole
wheat), lightly toasted

1. In a medium bowl, combine the ground chicken, bread crumbs or TVP, red bell pepper, green onions, green chilies, salt, if using, and ground black pepper. With lightly moistened hands, form the mixture into four 4-inch patties.
2. Prepare the grill or electric grilling machine for cooking.
3. If using a charcoal grill, place the patties over ashen coals on the hottest area of a lightly oiled grid for 1 to 2 minutes on each side to brown. Move the patties to a cooler part of the grill and continue to cook for another 3 to 4 minutes on each side, or until the meat is thoroughly cooked (no pink remains and the juices run clear) and the patties spring back to the touch. When the burgers are nearly done, toast the buns on the coolest part of the grill.
4. If using an electric grilling machine, grill the patties for about 4 minutes, or until the meat is thoroughly cooked (no pink remains and the juices run clear) and the patties spring back to the touch. While the burgers are cooking, toast the buns in a skillet lightly brushed with oil or toast in the grilling machine for about 1 minute after the meat has cooked.
5. Spread the buns with your favorite condiment or with Roasted Red Pepper Mayonnaise and top with lettuce and thinly sliced onions.

Preparation time: *10 minutes*
Cooking time: *8–12 minutes on a grill; about 4 minutes in an electric grilling machine*
Makes 4 servings

Nutritional Breakdown (per serving)

Calories: 426   Carbohydrates: 55 gm   Cholesterol: 52 mg   Saturated fat: 1 gm
Protein: 28 gm   Sodium: 183 mg   Fat: 10 gm   % calories fat: 21%

When preparing ground chicken (or any ground meat), be sure to wash your hands, cutting board, utensils, and any other surfaces touched by the raw food in hot, soapy water. Improper handling of raw poultry or meat at home is the cause of many food-borne illnesses each year. Also, make sure that all ground poultry or meat is cooked thoroughly, meaning there is no pink remaining and the juices run clear. (For more tips on safe handling and healthier cooking, see pages 23–24.)

Deluxe Turkey Burgers ♡

Turkey burgers never tasted so good as with the addition of apples, parsley, and bread crumbs or TVP (textured vegetable [soy] protein), which also helps reduce the amount of fat. The Onion-Dill Sauce (page 53) goes well with these burgers.

³/₄ pound ground, skinless turkey breast
¼ cup finely chopped sweet apple
¼ cup finely chopped fresh parsley
¼ cup seasoned bread crumbs or TVP (textured vegetable [soy] protein)

½ teaspoon salt (optional)
Reduced-fat Cheddar cheese (optional)
Canola oil for the grid, if using a grill
4 hamburger buns (preferably whole wheat), lightly toasted

1. In a medium bowl, combine the ground turkey, apple, parsley, bread crumbs or TVP, and salt, if using, and mix well. With lightly moistened hands, form the mixture into four 4-inch patties.
2. Prepare the grill or electric grilling machine for cooking.

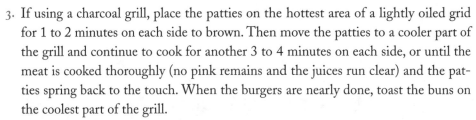

George Foreman's Knock-Out-the-Fat Barbecue and Grilling Cookbook

3. If using a charcoal grill, place the patties on the hottest area of a lightly oiled grid for 1 to 2 minutes on each side to brown. Then move the patties to a cooler part of the grill and continue to cook for another 3 to 4 minutes on each side, or until the meat is cooked thoroughly (no pink remains and the juices run clear) and the patties spring back to the touch. When the burgers are nearly done, toast the buns on the coolest part of the grill.

4. If using an electric grilling machine, grill the patties for about 4 minutes, or until cooked thoroughly (the juices run clear and no pink remains) and the patties spring back to the touch. While the burgers are cooking, toast the buns in a skillet lightly brushed with oil or toast in the grilling machine for about 1 minute after the meat is done.

5. Melt a slice of Cheddar cheese, if desired, on top of each patty toward the end of the cooking time.

6. Spread the buns with Onion-Dill Sauce, if using, and add other desired toppings, such as lettuce and thinly sliced tomatoes.

Preparation time: *10 minutes*
Cooking time: *8–12 minutes on a grill; about 4 minutes in an electric grilling machine*
Makes 4 servings

Nutritional Breakdown (per serving)

Calories: 435	*Carbohydrates: 56 gm*	*Cholesterol: 32 mg*	*Saturated fat: 2 gm*
Protein: 20 gm	*Sodium: 305 mg*	*Fat: 14 gm*	*% calories fat: 29%*

Nutribite

Turkey is a healthy substitute for ground beef when your taste buds are begging for a burger. Skinless ground turkey breast has a mere 3 grams of fat and only 129 calories per 4 ounces, versus 169 calories and 9 grams of fat found in 90 percent lean ground beef. These numbers, however, are based on ground turkey breast with no skin. You may need to ask your butcher to grind boneless, skinless breast meat or grind it yourself at home.

Philly Cheese Steak Sandwiches ♡

❋ Native to Philadelphia, these sandwiches are absolutely delicious, especially when served with the vegetable sauce. And who would believe they could boast the heart-healthy symbol!

Vegetable Sauce

1 tablespoon butter
1 tablespoon extra-virgin olive oil
1/2 cup thinly sliced onion
1/2 cup thinly sliced red bell pepper
1/2 cup thinly sliced green bell pepper

1 garlic clove, minced
6 mushrooms, thinly sliced
1 cup chopped tomato
1/2 teaspoon freshly ground black pepper

Cheese Steak Sandwich

1 pound thinly sliced sirloin steak*
2 skewers soaked in water for 15–30
    minutes, if using a grill
Canola oil for the grid, if using a grill

4 hoagie or steak rolls, grilled
Salt and pepper to taste (optional)
1/2 cup grated reduced-fat Cheddar cheese

1. To make the Vegetable Sauce, melt the butter in a large skillet over medium-high heat. Add the oil, onion, bell peppers, and garlic, and cook for 8 minutes. Add the mushrooms and sauté for 2 minutes. Reduce the heat to low, and add the tomatoes and black pepper; sauté for about 5 more minutes, or until all the vegetables are soft and the tomatoes have a pastelike consistency.
2. Prepare the grill or electric grilling machine for cooking.
3. If using a grill, thread the beef strips on the skewers and place on an oiled grid over ashen coals for 4 to 5 minutes for medium rare to medium, turning occasionally. Cut the rolls in half, if needed, and grill by placing the cut side down on the coolest part of the grill for the last 2 minutes of grilling. Remove the steak and rolls from the grill, and season the steak with salt or pepper, if using.
4. If using an electric grilling machine, place the meat on a hot grill for 1 to 1½ minutes for medium rare. Cut the rolls in half, if needed. Place the rolls, 1 or 2 at a time,

* To aid in slicing meat more thinly, place it in the freezer 30 minutes first.

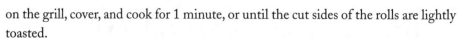

George Foreman's Knock-Out-the-Fat Barbecue and Grilling Cookbook

on the grill, cover, and cook for 1 minute, or until the cut sides of the rolls are lightly toasted.

5. To assemble the sandwich, divide the steak strips and vegetables into 4 portions and place the steak on the grilled rolls, spread the vegetables over the meat, and top each with about 2 tablespoons of the grated cheese.

Preparation time: *15 minutes*
Cooking time: *about 5 minutes using a grill; about 3 minutes using an electric grilling machine*
Makes 4 servings

Nutritional Breakdown (per serving)

Calories: 752	*Carbohydrates: 84 gm*	*Cholesterol: 93 mg*	*Saturated fat: 8 gm*
Protein: 49 gm	*Sodium: 901 mg*	*Fat: 24 gm*	*% calories fat: 29%*

Nutribite

When you opt to use cheese in a recipe or on a burger, keep in mind that Swiss cheese is 1 gram lower in fat than Cheddar, American, or Monterey Jack, with 8 grams of fat versus 9 grams in each ounce. Better yet are reduced-fat cheeses like Cheddar or Swiss with only 4 grams of fat per ounce, which are healthy choices if they are made with skim milk. Avoid brands that contain chemicals or unnatural substances.

Cherie's American Gyros with Cucumber-Yogurt Sauce

One of Cherie and her husband, John's, favorite food feasts is held at Seattle's Greek Festival at the Greek Orthodox Church. Gyros are always their favorite choice. This recipe is her version of the traditional Greek gyro, and John thinks hers are the best.

Mint Marinade

Juice of ½ orange

¼ cup light soy sauce or tamari

1 tablespoon raspberry vinegar

1 tablespoon extra-virgin olive oil

1 tablespoon chopped fresh mint, or
    ½ tablespoon dried

¼ teaspoon freshly ground black pepper

Grilled Lamb

1–1½ pounds lean loin lamb, pounded and
    thinly sliced*

4 pita pockets, cut in half

4 bamboo skewers soaked in water 15–30
    minutes, if using a grill

Canola oil, if using a grill

Cucumber-Yogurt Sauce

½ cup minced cucumber, seeded

½ cup plain low-fat yogurt

2 tablespoons chopped fresh mint, or
    1 tablespoon dried

2 tablespoons chopped fresh cilantro, or
    1 tablespoon dried

2 tablespoons chopped green onions

1 tablespoon fresh lime juice

1. To make the Mint Marinade, combine all the ingredients in a medium bowl and mix well.
2. Put the sliced lamb in the marinade, cover, and refrigerate for 1 to 2 hours.
3. While the lamb is marinating, prepare the Cucumber-Yogurt Sauce. Place all the ingredients in the bowl of a blender or food processor with a steel blade and process for about 1 minute, or until combined well.

* To help slice meat more thinly, place it in the freezer for 30 minutes first. And if you want tender meat, always slice it against the grain.

4. Prepare the grill or electric grilling machine for cooking.

5. If using a charcoal grill, thread the lamb onto skewers and place on an oiled grid above ashen coals. Cook for 2 minutes, baste with the reserved marinade, and turn, and cook for another 2 minutes for medium rare.

5. If using an electric grilling machine, place the lamb on a hot grill, drizzle a bit of the marinade over the top, and cook for about 1 minute and 15 seconds for medium rare.

7. To assemble the gyros, place several strips of lamb in each pita pocket half, spoon 2 to 4 tablespoons Cucumber-Yogurt Sauce over the meat, and serve hot.

Preparation time: *15 minutes*
Cooking time: *4 minutes on a grill; 1¼ minutes in an electric grilling machine*
Makes 1½ cups sauce: *8 half-pocket sandwich servings or 4 whole-pocket sandwiches*

Nutritional Breakdown (based on 1 half-pocket serving with 2 tablespoons sauce)

Calories: 184	*Carbohydrates: 18 gm*	*Cholesterol: 37 mg*	*Saturated fat: 2 gm*
Protein: 15 gm	*Sodium: 351 mg*	*Fat: 5 gm*	*% calories fat: 27%*

Garden Burgers ♡

Veggie burgers are often my first choice in a sandwich. Especially when I'm in training, I really watch the amount of red meat I eat and I'll choose vegetarian meals for several weeks, even a month at a time, to keep my body in top shape. If you want to eat like a champ, make some of your days, weeks, or months vegetarian, too. The Garden Burger is a good place to start. Served with your favorite barbecue sauce or mustard, lettuce, and tomato, the only thing you'll miss out on is the extra fat and cholesterol.

2 tablespoons extra-virgin olive oil
½ cup chopped onion
½ cup chopped zucchini
½ cup coarsely chopped water chestnuts
¼ cup chopped mushrooms
¼ cup chopped fresh parsley
2 garlic cloves, minced
1½ cups hot water
2 tablespoons tamari or light soy sauce
1½ cups TVP (textured vegetable [soy] protein)

½ cup cooked garbanzo beans (chick peas)
½ cup ground sunflower seeds
2 tablespoons plain nonfat yogurt
½ teaspoon coarsely ground black pepper
½ teaspoon ground cumin
¼ teaspoon cayenne pepper
2 egg whites
½ cup bread crumbs
Canola oil for the grid, if using a grill
8 hamburger buns (preferably whole wheat), toasted

1. In a medium skillet, heat the oil over medium-high heat; add the onion, zucchini, water chestnuts, mushrooms, parsley, and garlic. Sauté until the vegetables are tender, about 10 minutes.

2. While the vegetables are cooking, heat the water in a small saucepan over high heat. Remove the saucepan from the heat and add the tamari.

3. Add the TVP to the bowl of a food processor or blender, and add the water mixture. Let it sit for about 10 minutes until the TVP is hydrated. Add the garbanzo beans, sunflower seeds, yogurt, black pepper, cumin, cayenne pepper, and egg whites; blend until smooth.

4. Scoop the TVP mixture into a large mixing bowl, and stir in the sautéed vegetables, mixing well.

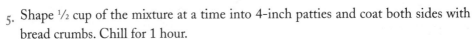

5. Shape ½ cup of the mixture at a time into 4-inch patties and coat both sides with bread crumbs. Chill for 1 hour.

6. Prepare the grill or electric grilling machine for cooking.

7. If using a charcoal grill, place the burgers on an oiled grid above ashen coals and cook for 3 to 4 minutes on each side. Toast the buns on the coolest part of the grill for the last 2 minutes.

8. If using an electric grilling machine, place the burgers 4 at a time on a hot grill and cook for about 8 minutes. Toast the buns in a skillet lightly brushed with oil or in the grilling machine for about 1 minute after the meat is done.

Preparation time: *about 20 minutes*
Cooking time: *6–8 minutes on a grill; 6–8 minutes in an electric grilling machine*
Makes 8 servings

Nutritional Breakdown (per serving)

Calories: 348	*Carbohydrates: 34 gm*	*Cholesterol: 0 mg*	*Saturated fat: 1.5 gm*
Protein: 30 gm	*Sodium: 435 mg*	*Fat: 11 gm*	*% calories fat: 28%*

Nutribite

Plain nonfat yogurt is a versatile food for healthy cooking. It mixes well with mayonnaise and blends well in creamy salad dressings. In addition, it makes an excellent base for sauces such as the Cucumber-Yogurt Sauce (page 59). Plus it offers another nutritional benefit, acidophilus—the good bacterial culture that's important for a healthy digestive tract.

CHAPTER EIGHT

BEEF

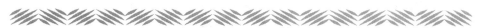

BEEF WAS THE STAR OF OUTDOOR COOKING LONG BEFORE THE West was won. Though we are more aware now of beef's high fat content (18 to 41 percent fat versus 20 to 25 percent in chicken, for example), it's still a popular choice for backyard parties, picnics, and family grilling.

Tender cuts of beef from the loin, such as tenderloin, top sirloin, porterhouse, T-bone, New York strip, and filet mignon, as well as steaks from the prime rib such as rib eye and Delmonico, can be cooked directly over the heat, and because the meat's marbled with fat, it stays moist and juicy. Other cuts from the chuck, rib, cross rib, shank, flank, or leg need marinating to tenderize them, and should be cooked over a drip pan with indirect heat.

Buy the leanest cuts, such as flank or round steak, and trim away all visible fat. Keep the portions small, as the USDA Food Guide Pyramid suggests: around 3 ounces per serving. Also, strive to eat red meat only once in a while, rather than often. A Harvard University study found that people who ate a main dish of red meat daily were 250 percent more likely to develop colon cancer than those eating meat less than once a month. Be aware, too, that red meat is high in heme-type iron. Though an important consideration for children and women of childbearing age, excess iron consumption in men and postmenopausal women can lead to heart disease and premature aging.

For the healthiest meat, look for beef that has been naturally raised. *Natural* indicates that the animals were raised without the assistance of growth stimulants, hormones, antibiotics, steroids, or any other drugs. It should also mean the animals have been fed an *organic* diet—feed that's free of pesticides—and that they've been able to roam for their food rather than being confined to pens. Such practices result in healthier animals, which in turn produce healthier meat. Read labels and look for those that say *grown naturally,* or ask your grocer to carry these products in your market.

TIPS FOR GRILLING AND BARBECUING BEEF

1. Grill all beef over medium to medium-low temperature coals. Coals that are too hot can cause beef to overcook, which makes steaks tough and less flavorful. Beef is the most flavorful when grilled just to the proper doneness.

2. Determine the doneness of steaks by making a small slit near the bone and checking the color; for boneless cuts, make a small slit near the center or check the temperature with a meat thermometer.
   - Medium rare: center is very pink and slightly brown toward the exterior; 130°F to 135°F
   - Medium: center is light pink and outer portion is brown; 140°F to 145°F
   - Medium well done: mostly brown throughout; 150°F to 155°F
   - Well done: uniformly brown throughout; 160°F to 170°F

3. To keep the flavor, use long-handled tongs for turning steaks and a long-handled spatula for burgers. Piercing the meat with a fork when turning allows the flavorful juices to escape.

4. Beef ribs, short ribs, and brisket are best for barbecuing. Beef ribs are tender enough that they can be cooked directly over heat, but short ribs should always be cooked slowly over a drip pan.

5. After marinating raw meat, always cook the marinating sauce well before serving.

6. Always wash the platter you used to carry raw meat to your grill before serving cooked meat or any other food on it.

Grilled Steak Strips over Santa Fe Salad

If you've planned a busy day and have little time to spend in the kitchen, this multi-textured Southwestern salad can be made in just minutes, but it will taste like you've been in the kitchen a lot longer. This salad goes well with cornbread and corn muffins, or with tortilla chips and fresh salsa (see South of the Border Salsa, page 66).

1 pound boneless beef sirloin steak (turkey or chicken can be substituted)
Canola oil to brush the grid, if using a grill
Salt and pepper to taste (optional)
1 cup cubed reduced-fat Cheddar cheese
1 cup chopped red bell pepper
1 cup chopped green bell pepper
1 cup cooked black beans

1 cup fresh corn cut off the cob (frozen or canned corn, drained, can be substituted)
½ cup chopped jicama (optional)
1 medium onion, finely chopped
4 cups lettuce, washed, dried, and torn into bite-size pieces (a combination of green leaf and iceberg is good)
½ bag (about 6 ounces) corn tortilla chips, crumbled

Creamy Salsa Dressing
¼ cup plus 2 tablespoons fresh or prepared salsa

¼ cup reduced-fat mayonnaise
1 tablespoon fresh lime juice (optional)

Garnish
Fresh sprigs of cilantro

1. Prepare the grill or electric grilling machine for cooking.
2. If using a charcoal grill, place the steak on a lightly oiled grid over ashen coals. Grill the steak for 15 to 18 minutes for medium rare to medium doneness, turning occasionally. Remove from the grill, season to taste, and set aside to cool. When cool enough to handle, slice the steak across the grain into ⅛-inch-thick strips, season to taste, and set aside.

3. If using an electric grilling machine, grill the steak for $4^1/_2$ to 5 minutes for medium rare, $5^1/_2$ minutes for medium, or 6 minutes for well done, for each 1 inch of thickness. Remove from the grill, season to taste, and set aside to cool. When cool enough to handle, slice the steak across the grain into $1/_8$-inch-thick strips, season to taste, and set aside.

4. In a large salad bowl, place the cheese, peppers, black beans, corn, jicama, if using, and onion. Add the lettuce just before tossing.

5. To make the dressing, combine the salsa, mayonnaise, and lime juice, if using, in a small bowl, stirring until well combined. Cover and refrigerate until ready to use.

6. To assemble the salad, add the lettuce and toss with the Creamy Salsa Dressing. Serve the salad on 4 individual plates. Sprinkle $1/_4$ of the crumbled chips over each salad and decoratively arrange the steak strips on top. Garnish with cilantro sprigs.

Preparation time: *10–15 minutes*
Cooking time: *15–18 minutes for medium rare on a grill; $4^1/_2$–5 minutes for medium rare in an electric grilling machine*
Makes 4 servings

Nutritional Breakdown (per serving)

Calories: 673	Carbohydrates: 58 gm	Cholesterol: 100 mg	Saturated fat: 10 gm
Protein: 44 gm	Sodium: 512 mg	Fat: 31 gm	% calories fat: 40%

South of the Border Salsa ♡

3 Anaheim chili peppers (mild green) *$3/_4$ cup chopped fresh cilantro*
3 large or 6 small ripe tomatoes *$1/_4$ cup seasoned rice vinegar*
1 large firm cucumber, peeled and chopped *3 tablespoons fresh lime juice*
1 white onion, chopped *1 teaspoon ground cumin*
3 garlic cloves, minced *Salt and pepper to taste (optional)*

1. Roast the chili peppers (see page 50).
2. Cut the tomatoes in half, remove the seeds and excess juice, and chop.
3. In a large bowl, combine the chili peppers, tomatoes, cucumber, and onion. Add the garlic, and stir in the cilantro, vinegar, lime juice, and cumin. Add salt and pepper, if using, and chill until ready to serve.

Preparation time: *10 minutes*
Cooking time: *about 10 minutes for roasting peppers*
Makes 4 cups

Nutritional Breakdown (¼ cup per serving)

Calories: 29   *Carbohydrates: 7 gm*   *Cholesterol: 0 mg*   *Saturated fat: 0 gm*

Protein: 1 gm   *Sodium: 7 mg*   *Fat: 0 gm*   *% calories fat: 0*

Grilled Steak and Onion Salad with Tarragon-Dijon Dressing

If your taste buds yearn for steak, but you're trying to cut back on the amount of red meat in your diet, this salad is a perfect alternative. Four ounces of steak is quite filling when combined with lots of greens. Served with crusty bread, this main-course salad makes a complete meal.

1 pound boneless beef sirloin steak
Canola oil to brush the grid, if using a grill
Salt and pepper to taste (optional)
1 large onion, cut in small cubes
1–2 bamboo skewers soaked in water for 15–30 minutes, if using a grill

½ head romaine lettuce, washed, dried, and torn in bite-size pieces
½ head green or red leaf lettuce, washed, dried, and torn in bite-size pieces
1 cup baby field greens (optional)

Tarragon-Dijon Dressing

¼ cup extra-virgin olive oil
¼ cup fresh lemon juice
2 teaspoons Dijon mustard

2 teaspoons fresh tarragon or 1 teaspoon dried
½ teaspoon salt (optional)

1. Prepare the grill or electric grilling machine for cooking.
2. If using a charcoal grill, place the steak on a lightly oiled grid over ashen coals. Grill the steak for 15 to 18 minutes for medium rare to medium doneness, turning occasionally. Place onion skewers on grill 5 to 7 minutes before the steak is done, brush

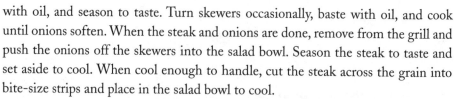
with oil, and season to taste. Turn skewers occasionally, baste with oil, and cook until onions soften. When the steak and onions are done, remove from the grill and push the onions off the skewers into the salad bowl. Season the steak to taste and set aside to cool. When cool enough to handle, cut the steak across the grain into bite-size strips and place in the salad bowl to cool.

3. If using an electric grilling machine, grill the steak for $4\frac{1}{4}$ to 5 minutes for medium rare or $5\frac{1}{2}$ minutes for medium doneness. Remove from the grill, season to taste, and set aside to cool. Place the onions on the grill, season to taste, and cook for about 3 minutes, or until softened. Remove and put the onions in the salad bowl to cool. When the steak is cool enough to handle, slice it across the grain into bite-size strips and place in the salad bowl to cool.

4. To make the dressing, in a small bowl, whisk together the olive oil, lemon juice, Dijon mustard, tarragon, and salt, if using.

5. Add the lettuce to the salad bowl when the onions and steak have cooled. Toss with the dressing and serve chilled.

Preparation time: *15 minutes*

Cooking time: *15–18 minutes for medium rare on a grill; $4\frac{1}{4}$–5 minutes for medium rare plus about 3 minutes for the onions in an electric grilling machine*

Makes 4 servings

Nutritional Breakdown (per serving)

Calories: 410	Carbohydrates: 19 gm	Cholesterol: 75 mg	Saturated fat: 6 gm
Protein: 29 gm	Sodium: 124 mg	Fat: 24 gm	% calories fat: 52%

Nutribite

Serving onions with a high-fat food like red meat is heart-smart. Whether onions are cooked or served raw, studies have shown that they have the ability to lower blood cholesterol and to bring cholesterol back down when they are eaten with a high-fat meal. In addition, onions raise HDL, the beneficial cholesterol, and can help to lower blood pressure. For a thankful heart, serve plenty of onions every time you serve red meat.

George's Sausage Texas-Style

Sporting true Southern flavor, this sizzling beef sausage is good served for break-fast with fresh salsa and a sautéed vegetable and egg scramble. (This recipe is from Cherie's book *The Healthy Gourmet*, published by Clarkson Potter.)

1 slightly beaten egg white
⅓ cup finely chopped onion
¼ cup seasoned bread crumbs or TVP (tex-tured vegetable [soy] protein)
¼ cup diced green chili peppers
1 large garlic clove, finely minced
2 tablespoons snipped fresh cilantro

1 tablespoon apple cider vinegar
1½ teaspoons chili powder
¼ teaspoon salt (optional)
Pinch cayenne pepper
½ pound extra-lean ground beef (90 per-cent lean contains the least fat)
Canola oil for the grid, if using a grill

1. In a medium mixing bowl, combine the egg white, onion, bread crumbs or TVP, chili peppers, garlic, cilantro, vinegar, chili powder, salt, if using, and cayenne pep-per. Add the ground beef and mix well.
2. Shape the mixture into eight 3-inch patties.
3. Prepare the grill or electric grilling machine for cooking.
4. If using a charcoal grill, oil the grid and place the patties over ashen coals and cook them for about 5 minutes per side. The patties should look like well-done ham-burgers, with no pink and with clear juices.
5. If using an electric grilling machine, place the patties on a hot grill and cook for 4 to 5 minutes. The patties should look like well-done hamburgers, with no pink and with clear juices.

Preparation time: *10 minutes*
Cooking time: *about 10 minutes on a grill; 4–5 minutes in an electric grilling machine*
Makes 4 servings (2 patties each)

Nutritional Breakdown (per serving)

Calories: 151	*Carbohydrates: 8 gm*	*Cholesterol: 35 mg*	*Saturated fat: 35 gm*
Protein: 13 gm	*Sodium: 307 mg*	*Fat: 7 gm*	*% calories fat: 44%*

Nutribite ⋙

To make fat-reduced sausage patties and burgers, you can save a considerable amount of fat and calories by choosing 90 percent lean ground beef. Ninety percent lean has 9 grams of fat, with 4 of those grams being saturated. This makes it a healthier choice than 73 percent lean beef, which has 18 grams of fat with 7 saturated-fat grams.

Herbed Steak Dijon

⋙ Top sirloin is featured here, but you can easily use T-bone, porterhouse, rib eye, club, New York, or filet mignon. Keep in mind that the USDA, ADA, and many other nutrition-conscious organizations recommend that we eat no more than 3 to 4 ounces of meat per serving. However, if you're like me, when you want a grilled steak, you want an ample portion. Therefore, Cherie and I have recommended larger servings in this recipe. But if you're watching the fat in your diet more closely, you can cut the steak portions down as desired.

4 garlic cloves, minced
1 tablespoon water
2 tablespoons Dijon mustard
1 teaspoon dried basil
½ teaspoon dried thyme

½ teaspoon freshly ground black pepper
4 top sirloin steaks (8–10 ounces each), well
   trimmed, cut 1 inch thick
Canola oil for the grid, if using a grill
Salt and pepper to taste (optional)

1. In a small saucepan, combine the garlic and water, and cook on high heat for 2 minutes. Stir in the mustard, basil, thyme, and pepper, and mix well. Remove from the heat and set aside.
2. Spread the herbed mustard over the steaks on both sides.
3. Prepare the grill or electric grilling machine for cooking.
4. If using a charcoal grill, place the steaks on an oiled grid over ashen coals. Grill for 15 to 18 minutes for medium rare to medium, turning occasionally, for each

1 inch of thickness. Remove from the grill, and season with salt and pepper to taste, if using.

5. If using an electric grilling machine, grill the steak for approximately 4½ to 5 minutes for medium rare for each 1 inch of thickness. Remove and add salt and pepper to taste, if using.

Preparation time: *5 minutes*
Cooking time: *15–18 minutes for medium rare on a grill; 4½–5 minutes for medium rare in an electric grilling machine*
Makes 4 servings

Nutritional Breakdown (per serving)

Calories: 1021	*Carbohydrates: 11 gm*	*Cholesterol: 378 mg*	*Saturated fat: 21 gm*
Protein: 129 gm	*Sodium: 469 mg*	*Fat: 51 gm*	*% calories fat: 46%*

Grilled Steak with Ginger-Soy Marinade

This Asian-influenced marinade gives grilled steak a new dimension of flavor. It goes well with garlic-roasted new potatoes and gingered carrots. Especially tasty for a late-summer or autumn evening steak grill, ginger is used traditionally in Asian cooking as a "warming food." It can help relieve the feeling of inner chill.

1 recipe Ginger-Soy Marinade (page 36)   *Canola oil for the grid, if using a grill*
4 sirloin steaks or any steak of your choice
   (allow 6–8 ounces per serving)

1. Prepare the marinade. Pour it over the steak and refrigerate for 3 hours to overnight. Let the steaks stand at room temperature for 30 minutes before grilling.
2. Prepare the grill or electric grilling machine for cooking.
3. If using a charcoal grill, place the steaks on an oiled grid over ashen coals. Grill for 15 to 18 minutes for medium rare to medium for each 1 inch of thickness, turning once.

4. If using an electric grilling machine, grill 4½ to 5 minutes for medium rare for each 1 inch of thickness.

Preparation time: *5 minutes for marinade*
Cooking time: *15–18 minutes for medium rare on the grill; 4½–5 minutes for medium rare in an electric grilling machine*
Makes 4 servings

Nutritional Breakdown (per serving, based on 6 ounces of sirloin steak)

Calories: 468	*Carbohydrates: 10 gm*	*Cholesterol: 113 mg*	*Saturated fat: 8 gm*
Protein: 39 gm	*Sodium: 708 mg*	*Fat: 29 gm*	*% calories fat: 55%*

Flank Steak Strips
with Hot Honey-Molasses Sauce

≫ Looking for an impressive dish for your next backyard barbecue? With this sweet, hot, and sassy sauce, flank steak never tasted so good. You'll want to freeze what's left for your next party—if there is any, that is.

Hot Honey-Molasses Sauce

2 tablespoons extra-virgin olive oil	*1 cup honey*
¼ cup minced onion	*¼ cup blackstrap molasses*
¼ cup minced green bell pepper	*2 tablespoons yellow mustard*
2 garlic cloves, minced	*1¼ teaspoon red pepper flakes*
1 (10¾ ounce) can tomato puree	*1 teaspoon chili powder*
1 cup apple cider vinegar	

Flank Steak

1½ pounds flank steak, trimmed of all visible fat and connective tissue	*Canola oil for the grid, if using a grill*

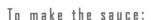
To make the sauce:

1. In a medium saucepan, heat the oil over medium-high heat, and add the onion, bell pepper, and garlic. Sauté for about 10 minutes, or until tender.
2. Add the tomato puree, apple cider vinegar, honey, blackstrap molasses, mustard, red pepper flakes, and chili powder. Reduce the heat to low, and simmer for 30 to 40 minutes, or until the sauce has thickened.

To prepare the steak:

1. Prepare the grill or electric grilling machine for cooking.
2. If using a charcoal grill, oil the grid and place it above ashen coals. Sear the meat over the hottest part of the coals, about 2 minutes per side. Then move it to a cooler area and cook to medium rare for about 3 to 4 minutes per side. Brush the sauce on the steak just before turning and then brush the top side with sauce.
3. If using an electric grilling machine, place the flank steak on a hot grill and cook for about 3 minutes for medium rare. After $1^{1}/_{2}$ minutes, brush the sauce on the top side.
4. To serve, slice the flank steak into thin strips against the grain. Spoon some of the Hot Honey-Molasses Sauce over the top and serve immediately.

Preparation time: *10 minutes*
Cooking time: *40–50 minutes for the sauce; 10–12 minutes for medium rare on a grill; about 3 minutes for medium rare in an electric grilling machine*
Makes 4 servings and about 4 cups of sauce

Nutritional Breakdown (per serving with about ¼ cup of sauce)

Calories: 463	*Carbohydrates: 26 gm*	*Cholesterol: 75 mg*	*Saturated fat: 6 gm*
Protein: 47 gm	*Sodium: 503 mg*	*Fat: 20 gm*	*% calories fat: 38%*

Lean, Mean Steak Fajitas

Mexican-style fajitas are rapidly becoming as popular as tacos in American homes and restaurants. Fajitas are a great way to stretch one 16-ounce steak into a meal for 4 to 6 people, and a delicious way to get everyone to eat more vegetables. Remember that the steak strips should marinate for 4 to 6 hours before grilling for the most flavor, but if you're in a hurry, even an hour will help. If you have only minutes to prepare the meal, cut the steak in strips and squeeze lime juice over them. Grill the steak strips and then season to taste.

Marinade

¼ cup fresh lime juice
2 tablespoons Worcestershire sauce
1 tablespoon canola oil
½ teaspoon freshly grated lemon zest
½ teaspoon freshly ground black pepper

¼ teaspoon paprika
¼ teaspoon ground cumin
¼ teaspoon ground chili powder
1 garlic clove, finely minced

Steak Fajitas

1¼ pounds boneless top sirloin (chicken can be substituted), cut against the grain into ½-inch strips
2 medium onions, cut into slices
1 red bell pepper, cut into strips
1 green bell pepper, cut into strips

Salt and pepper to taste (optional)
4–6 flour tortillas
Canola oil for the grid, if using a grill
8–12 skewers soaked in water for 15–30 minutes, if using a grill

Topping Options

Salsa (page 66)
Reduced-fat Cheddar or Monterey Jack cheese, grated

Guacamole
Fresh cilantro, chopped
Reduced-fat sour cream

1. To make the marinade, place all the ingredients in a medium bowl and stir until well blended.
2. Trim the fat from the steak and cut across the grain into ½-inch strips.

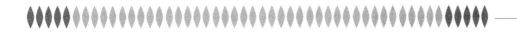
3. Pour the marinade into a large resealable plastic bag and add the steak strips. Seal the bag and turn several times so all the steak strips are covered with the marinade. Marinate in the refrigerator for 4 to 6 hours. Drain and reserve the marinade.

4. Prepare the grill or electric grilling machine for cooking.

5. If using a charcoal grill, thread the peppers onto skewers and place on an oiled grid over ashen coals. Grill for 15 to 18 minutes. Thread the onions onto skewers and grill for 12 to 15 minutes or until they are tender, turning once. Brush the vegetables with the reserved marinade occasionally. Thread the steak strips onto skewers. About 10 minutes before the vegetables are done, move them to a cooler part of the grid. Place the steak strips in the center of the grid and grill for 8 to 10 minutes for medium rare to medium doneness, turning once. Brush with the reserved marinade. Remove the steak strips and vegetables from the grill, season to taste, and remove from the skewers.

6. If using an electric grilling machine, add the peppers, drizzle a bit of marinade over the top, cover, and cook 5 to 6 minutes, or until tender. After about 2 minutes, add the onions, drizzle a bit of the marinade over the top, cover, and cook for 3 to 4 minutes, or until tender. About 1 to 1½ minutes before the vegetables are done, push them to the top of the grill and place the steak strips on the lower portion of the grill for 1 to 1½ minutes for medium rare. Remove, place the steak, onions, and bell peppers in individual serving bowls, and cover to keep warm.

7. While the steak and vegetables are cooking, warm the tortillas by covering tightly and placing them in a warm oven (250°F) for about 15 minutes.

8. Place a tortilla on each dinner plate. Serve the steak and vegetables family-style, allowing everyone to roll their own fajitas. Serve with salsa, cheese, guacamole, cilantro, or sour cream toppings.

Preparation time: *20 minutes*
Cooking time: *15–18 minutes on a grill; 5–6 minutes in an electric grilling machine*
Makes 4–6 servings

Nutritional Breakdown (per serving)

Calories: 357	*Carbohydrates: 32 gm*	*Cholesterol: 63 mg*	*Saturated fat: 4 gm*
Protein: 26 gm	*Sodium: 273 mg*	*Fat: 13 gm*	*% calories fat: 34%*

Texas Barbecued Beef Ribs

The state of Texas has two champs—George Foreman and Texas barbecue sauce. The traditional Texas recipe is a very rich sauce that calls for a half cup of butter. Cherie and I have cut the fat to a quarter of that amount, and we've substituted honey and molasses for brown sugar. We think our sauce tastes no less rich and flavorful than the Texas original. But then, you'll have to judge for yourself.

Texas Barbecue Sauce

2 tablespoons butter

2 tablespoons canola oil

1 cup minced onion

1 cup minced celery

1 cup minced green pepper

2 tablespoons minced garlic

1¼ cups tomato puree

½ cup honey

¼ cup apple cider vinegar

¼ cup chicken stock

2 tablespoons Worcestershire sauce

2 tablespoons chili powder

1 teaspoon ground cumin

¼–½ teaspoon cayenne pepper, depending on hotness desired

¼ teaspoon freshly ground black pepper

2 bay leaves

Salt to taste (optional)

Beef Ribs

4 pounds trimmed beef ribs

Canola oil for the grid

1. To make the sauce, in a small skillet over medium-high heat, melt the butter, then add the oil, onion, celery, bell pepper, and garlic. Reduce the heat and sauté for about 10 minutes, or until the onion is translucent and the vegetables are soft.

2. Transfer the vegetable mixture to a nonaluminum saucepan, add the remaining ingredients and slowly simmer for about 30 minutes, stirring frequently so the sauce doesn't burn. Allow the sauce to sit at room temperature for at least 1 hour so the flavors can meld, then remove the bay leaves. If time allows, make the sauce the day before and store, covered, in the refrigerator. It's even more flavorful the next day.

3. Prepare the grill for cooking. (Beef ribs don't cook well on an electric grilling machine.)

4. If using a charcoal grill, place the ribs on an oiled grid directly over ashen coals and brown on both sides, about 3 minutes per side. Turn often and baste with sauce

when ribs are about half done. They are done in about 15 minutes, when nearly black on the outside.

Preparation time: *15–20 minutes*
Cooking time: *about 40 minutes for the sauce; about 15 minutes for the ribs*
Makes 4 servings

Nutritional Breakdown (per serving)

Calories: 1274	*Carbohydrates: 55 gm*	*Cholesterol: 277 mg*	*Saturated fat: 28 gm*
Protein: 108 gm	*Sodium: 750 mg*	*Fat: 69 gm*	*% calories fat: 49%*

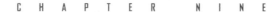

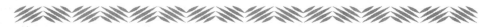

FISH AND SEAFOOD

FISH AND SEAFOOD ARE EXCELLENT CHOICES FOR GRILLING AND barbecuing, as they lend themselves well to different marinades, sauces, and dry rubs. Relatively low-fat, low-cholesterol protein sources, they are among the best providers of omega-3 fatty acids—the good fats. Fish and seafood have enough of the good oils to stay succulent and juicy on the grill. Using a hot fire will seal in the juices.

Research indicates that the omega-3 fats in fish help in preventing heart disease, are associated with clean arteries, and aid in the prevention of fatty degeneration. Studies show that eating fish two or more times per week may provide some of the cardiovascular benefits that have been observed in Eskimos, a population in which heart disease is notably rare. Omega-3s may also help to lower blood pressure and prevent cancer.

High-fat, cold-water fish, such as salmon, sardines, mackerel, tuna, and trout, offer the highest amount of these beneficial fats. And the highest concentration of these oils can be found just under the skin, especially behind the gills, around the fins, and in the belly region.

Amid the craze to avoid all fat in our diet, it is important to remember that some fats, the good ones like the omega-3 fatty acids found in fish and certain oils, are not only important for thick, shining hair and moist, supple skin, but are essential for overall health.

We suggest that you eat more fish and seafood. I do, especially when I'm in training. My favorites are catfish and swordfish, and I'm sure you'll agree that George's Catfish Fillets with Sesame Crust (page 92) and Ginger-Lime Swordfish (page 83) are the best.

TIPS FOR GRILLING AND BARBECUING FISH

1. Use a hinged grill basket to keep delicate fillets or whole fish intact as you turn. Place the basket on the grill, and oil and heat it up a bit before placing the fish inside.

2. Cook fish or seafood 4 to 6 inches from the heat, turning only once and brushing occasionally with oil or marinade to prevent drying.

3. Be careful not to overcook fish as it will become tough and dry.

4. Don't use leftover marinade from raw fish or seafood on your food unless it has been thoroughly heated first.

5. A general rule for cooking fish is to allow about 10 minutes of cooking time on the grill for each 1 inch of thickness. Allow about 5 minutes for each 1 inch of thickness when using an electric grilling machine.

6. Always wash the platter you used to carry raw fish to your grill before serving cooked fish or any other food on it.

7. To test for doneness, press the flesh of the fish with your fingertips. When the fish is done, it is "just firm"—raw is soft and overdone is hard and firm.

8. When the fish is done, serve it immediately on hot plates. It looks at its prettiest for about 5 minutes after being removed from the grill.

Grilled Salmon Steaks with Tarragon Sauce

Tarragon, with its sweet licorice flavor, makes a flavorful dry rub for fresh salmon, and it is an excellent addition to fish sauce. We suggest serving this salmon with a fresh green salad, lightly steamed vegetables such as green beans and carrots julienne, and lemon-zested brown rice.

4 salmon steaks (¹⁄₃ to ¹⁄₂ pound each)
2 tablespoons dried tarragon
Reduced-fat mayonnaise for coating the
    salmon, about 1 tablespoon per serving

Canola oil for brushing the grid, if using a
    grill
Salt and pepper to taste
Lemon wedges

1. Rinse the salmon steaks and pat dry. Sprinkle tarragon on both sides of the fish, pressing or rubbing gently to make sure it sticks. Lightly coat each steak with a bit of mayonnaise to prevent drying, being careful not to remove the tarragon.
2. Prepare the grill or electric grilling machine for cooking.
3. If using a charcoal grill, place the salmon steaks on an oiled grid directly over ashen coals. Allow 10 minutes of cooking time for each 1 inch of thickness. (A salmon steak is typically 1¹⁄₄ inches thick, in which case allow 12 to 13 minutes.) For a 1¹⁄₄-inch steak, cook for 6 minutes, and then turn and cook for another 6 to 7 minutes, or until the salmon is opaque and starts to flake. It should be firm yet moist. Be careful not to overcook or it will become dry and tough.
4. If using an electric grilling machine, place the salmon steaks on a hot grill for about 5 minutes, or until the fish is opaque and starts to flake. It should be firm yet moist. Be careful not to overcook or it will become dry and tough.
5. Put the steaks on a warm platter, season to taste, and sprinkle with fresh lemon juice. Serve immediately with lemon wedges and Tarragon Sauce (page 81).

Preparation time: *5 minutes*
Cooking time: *12–13 minutes on a grill for 1¹⁄₄ inches thickness; about 5 minutes in an electric grilling machine*
Makes 4 servings

Tarragon Sauce

2 tablespoons plain low-fat yogurt
2 tablespoons reduced-fat mayonnaise

3 teaspoons fresh tarragon, or 1½ teaspoons
   dried
½ teaspoon Dijon mustard

Mix all the ingredients well in a medium bowl and refrigerate until ready to serve.

Preparation time: *5 minutes*
Makes 4 servings

Nutritional Breakdown (per serving with about 2 tablespoons of sauce)

Calories: 199	Carbohydrates: 1 gm	Cholesterol: 76 mg	Saturated fat: 1 gm
Protein: 29 gm	Sodium: 114 mg	Fat: 8 gm	% calories fat: 38%

Nutribite 〰️

Salmon is one of the best sources of omega-3 fatty acids—essential fatty acids that have been associated with clean arteries and freedom from fatty degeneration. Some of the most powerful health-enhancing effects of these oils revolve around two specific fatty acids, namely EPA (eicosapentaenoic acid) and DHA (docosahexaenoic acid). Studies show that these fatty acids can help prevent clumping of saturated fats (those that like to stick together), and they help keep saturated fatty acids and cholesterol dispersed. Research shows that omega-3 fatty acids also aid in reducing inflammation and may benefit rheumatoid arthritis sufferers.

Barbecued Salmon Fillet with Dill-Wine Baste

You don't have to live in the Pacific Northwest to enjoy delicious fresh salmon, but after having called that area home for more than a decade, Cherie thinks there's no place like it for the best salmon you've ever tasted. Still, regardless of where you live, you can enjoy barbecued salmon fillets hot off the grill.

Dill-Wine Baste

¼ cup extra-virgin olive oil
¼ cup white wine vinegar
¼ cup dry white wine
2 tablespoons dried dill

1 tablespoon freshly grated lemon zest
¼ teaspoon freshly ground black pepper
2 garlic cloves, finely chopped
Juice of ½ lemon

Grilled Salmon

1–1½ pounds salmon fillet

Canola oil for the grid, if using a grill

1. To make the baste, place all the ingredients in a medium bowl, mix well, and set aside.
2. Prepare the grill or electric grilling machine for cooking.
3. If using a charcoal grill, oil the grid and place it over ashen coals. Place the salmon skin side down over a drip pan for indirect cooking. Brush the flesh side of the salmon with the Dill-Wine Baste. Cover and cook for 10 to 20 minutes, or until the flesh just turns opaque in the center, basting 2 or 3 times while cooking. Or, if using a hinged basket, turn with flesh side down for the last 3–4 minutes.
4. If using an electric grilling machine, skin the salmon and cut it into 4 pieces. Brush both sides of the fish with the Dill-Wine Baste. Place the salmon fillets on a hot grill and cook for about 4 to 5 minutes, or until the flesh just turns opaque in the center, basting once or twice while cooking.
5. Remove from the grill and cut into 4 servings.

Preparation time: *10 minutes*
Cooking time: *10–20 minutes on a grill; 4–5 minutes in an electric grilling machine*
Makes 4 servings, 4–6 ounces each

Nutritional Breakdown (per serving)

Calories: 198	*Carbohydrates: 1 gm*	*Cholesterol: 57 mg*	*Saturated fat: 1 gm*
Protein: 22 gm	*Sodium: 75 mg*	*Fat: 11 gm*	*% calories fat: 49%*

Ginger-Lime Swordfish

Swordfish is one of my favorites because it's firm-fleshed and looks like a piece of meat. Melt-in-your-mouth-tender is the only way to describe this swordfish grill. Marinating it for 2 to 6 hours is the key to great flavor and tenderness. Add grilled vegetables and oven-roasted potatoes for a sensational meal.

Ginger-Lime Marinade

3 tablespoons canola oil
2 green onions, thinly sliced
¼ cup fresh lime juice

1 tablespoon grated ginger
Salt and pepper to taste (optional)

Grilled Swordfish

1–1½ pounds swordfish
Canola oil for the grid, if using a grill

Salt and pepper to taste (optional)

1. To make the marinade, in a small saucepan, heat the oil and green onions over medium heat for 2 minutes. Stir in the lime juice, grated ginger, and salt and pepper, if using, and cook for 1 more minute.
2. Place the fish in a shallow dish and pour the warm marinade over the top. Cover and place in the refrigerator for at least 2 hours, turning once after an hour. Let the fish stand at room temperature for 30 minutes before grilling.
3. Prepare the grill or electric grilling machine for cooking.

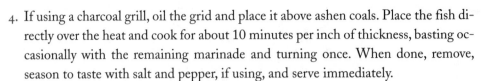
4. If using a charcoal grill, oil the grid and place it above ashen coals. Place the fish directly over the heat and cook for about 10 minutes per inch of thickness, basting occasionally with the remaining marinade and turning once. When done, remove, season to taste with salt and pepper, if using, and serve immediately.

5. If using an electric grilling machine, place the fish on a hot grill, drizzle a bit of marinade on top, and cook for 4 to 5 minutes for each inch of thickness. When done, remove, season to taste with salt and pepper, if using, and serve immediately.

Preparation time: *10 minutes*

Cooking time: *about 3 minutes for the marinade; 10 minutes on a grill; 4–5 minutes in an electric grilling machine*

Makes 4 servings

Nutritional Breakdown (per serving)

Calories: 188	Carbohydrates: 1 gm	Cholesterol: 45 mg	Saturated fat: 2 gm
Protein: 22 gm	Sodium: 102 mg	Fat: 10 gm	% calories fat: 48%

Swordfish is harvested in waters off New England in the summer and fall, and in the Gulf of Mexico, Florida, and Latin America in the winter. It's a popular fish for easy grilling, with a texture similar to steak. Its mild flavor picks up those of sauces and marinades very well.

Chef Mark's Tomato-Basil Halibut

Halibut is a firm-fleshed fish that looks somewhat like a cut of meat and has visual appeal to those who like eating thick cuts of meat. The Tomato-Basil Sauce is at its most flavorful in the summer and early fall, when vine-ripened tomatoes and garden-fresh basil are plentiful.

Marinade

¼ cup extra-virgin olive oil
1 tablespoon chopped fresh basil
¼ teaspoon freshly ground black pepper

Juice of ½ lemon
1 large garlic clove, minced

Grilled Halibut

1½–2 pounds fresh halibut steaks or fillets

Canola oil for the grid, if using a grill

Tomato-Basil Sauce

2 tablespoons extra-virgin olive oil
¼ cup chopped green onions
1 large garlic clove, minced

1 cup peeled and chopped vine-ripened tomatoes
2 heaping tablespoons chopped fresh basil
½ teaspoon freshly ground black pepper

Garnish

Fresh basil leaves

1. To prepare the marinade, combine all the ingredients in a shallow bowl and add the halibut, making sure that it fits snugly and that both sides of the fish are coated. Cover and refrigerate for 2 to 6 hours.
2. To prepare the Tomato-Basil Sauce, heat the oil in a small saucepan over medium heat and sauté the green onions and garlic for about 5 minutes. Add the tomatoes, basil, and black pepper, and simmer over low heat for about 10 minutes, or until the sauce thickens a bit.
3. Drain the halibut and reserve the marinade for basting. Allow the fish to sit at room temperature for 30 minutes before grilling.
4. Prepare the grill or electric grilling machine for cooking.

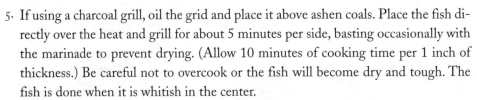

5. If using a charcoal grill, oil the grid and place it above ashen coals. Place the fish directly over the heat and grill for about 5 minutes per side, basting occasionally with the marinade to prevent drying. (Allow 10 minutes of cooking time per 1 inch of thickness.) Be careful not to overcook or the fish will become dry and tough. The fish is done when it is whitish in the center.

6. If using an electric grilling machine, place as many fish steaks or fillets on the grill as will fit at one time. Drizzle a bit of the marinade over the top and grill for about 3½ to 4 minutes, being careful not to overcook or the fish will become dry and tough. The fish is done when it is whitish in the center.

7. Place a halibut steak or fillet on each plate and spoon a bit of the Tomato-Basil Sauce on top. Garnish with a couple of basil leaves and serve immediately.

Preparation time: *15–20 minutes*

Cooking time: *15 minutes for the sauce; 10 minutes per inch on a grill; 3½–4 minutes in an electric grilling machine*

Makes 4 servings

Nutritional Breakdown (per serving)

Calories: 320	*Carbohydrates: 4 gm*	*Cholesterol: 55 mg*	*Saturated fat: 2 gm*
Protein: 36 gm	*Sodium: 190 mg*	*Fat: 17 gm*	*% calories fat: 50%*

Nutribite

Tomatoes and basil are good sources of a phytonutrient (*phyto* means "plant") known as monoterpene, which is a cancer-fighting antioxidant. Basil also contains compounds known to promote healing, reduce inflammation, and halt infection.

Albacore Tuna with Gingered Marinade

The Gingered Marinade makes fresh albacore tuna taste like it's been prepared in Hawaii. Serve this with fresh pineapple slices and pretend for just a moment that you can hear those tropical waves crashing on the shore.

Gingered Marinade

¼ cup fresh orange juice

¼ cup extra-virgin olive oil

¼ cup light soy sauce or tamari

¼ cup chopped green onions

1 tablespoon minced ginger

1 teaspoon minced garlic

¼ teaspoon freshly ground black pepper

¼ teaspoon cayenne pepper

Grilled Tuna

1–1½ pounds albacore tuna

Canola oil for the grid, if using a grill

1. To make the marinade, combine all the ingredients in a medium shallow dish. Add the tuna. Marinate in the refrigerator for 2 to 6 hours. Let sit at room temperature for 30 minutes before grilling.
2. Prepare the grill or electric grilling machine for cooking.
3. If using a charcoal grill, oil the grid and place it above ashen coals. Place the tuna directly above the heat and cook for about 10 minutes per inch of thickness, or until the center is opaque. Baste and turn once after 5 minutes.
4. If using an electric grilling machine, place the fish on a hot grill, drizzle a bit of the marinade over the top, and cook for 3½ to 4 minutes, or until the fish is opaque in the center of the thickest part.

Preparation: *5 minutes*
Cooking time: *10 minutes per inch on a grill; 3½–4 minutes in an electric grilling machine*
Makes 4 servings

Nutritional Breakdown (per serving)

Calories: 183	*Carbohydrates: 1 gm*	*Cholesterol: 49 mg*	*Saturated fat: 1 gm*
Protein: 26 gm	*Sodium: 352 mg*	*Fat: 8 gm*	*% calories fat: 39%*

Orange Roughy
with Zesty Fat-Free Marinade ♡

The lemon zest and tarragon add bursts of flavor to otherwise mild-flavored fish like orange roughy, whitefish, or turbot. If you're watching calories, the fat-free marinade lends exceptional flavor without added fat. And speaking of calories, orange roughy boasts only 70 calories per 3 ounces and contains 1 gram of fat, two reasons why this recipe earned the heart-healthy symbol. The remaining marinade is tasty thoroughly heated and served over brown rice.

1 recipe Zesty Fat-Free Marinade (page 33)
4 fillets orange roughy or any other firm-fleshed white fish (4–6 ounces each)

Canola oil for the grid, if using a grill
Salt and pepper to taste (optional)

1. Marinate the fish for 2 to 6 hours in the refrigerator; remove and let stand at room temperature for 30 minutes before grilling. Reserve the marinade.
2. Prepare the grill or electric grilling machine for cooking.
3. If using a charcoal grill, oil the grid and place it above ashen coals. Place the fish directly over the heat and cook for about 6 minutes (about 3 minutes per side), or until the fish is milky white in the center, basting occasionally with the remaining marinade. When done, remove from the grill, season to taste with salt and pepper, if using, and serve immediately.
4. If using an electric grilling machine, place the fish on a hot grill, drizzle a bit of the marinade on top, close the lid, and cook for about 3 minutes, or until the fish is milky white in the center. When done, remove from the grill, season to taste with salt and pepper, if using, and serve immediately.

Preparation time: *10 minutes*
Cooking time: *about 6 minutes on a grill; about 3 minutes using an electric grilling machine*
Makes 4 servings

Nutritional Breakdown (per serving)

Calories: 83	*Carbohydrates: 1 gm*	*Cholesterol: 22 mg*	*Saturated fat: 0*
Protein: 16 gm	*Sodium: 70 mg*	*Fat: 1 gm*	*% calories fat: 9%*

Grilled Flounder
with Dill-Wine Dry Rub ♡

Fish often gets dry and tough when cooked, but the flounder we made was so moist it was hard to believe it was fish. The dry rub adds zesty flavor to otherwise quite mild-flavored fish. (Not all dry rubs are free of liquid. Here, a bit of wine and lemon juice are added to facilitate spreading the rub.)

Dill-Wine Dry Rub

Juice of ½ lemon
2 tablespoons dry white wine
2 tablespoons chopped fresh dill, or
    1 tablespoon dried

2 teaspoons paprika
¼ teaspoon freshly ground black pepper
1 garlic clove, minced

Grilled Flounder

1–1½ pounds flounder or any other firm-
    fleshed white fish

Canola oil for the grid, if using a grill

1. To make the dry rub, combine all ingredients in a small bowl and mix well.
2. Wash the fish and pat dry. Spoon some of the dry rub over the fish and rub it into the flesh on both sides. Place the fish on a plate, cover, and refrigerate for 1 to 2 hours.

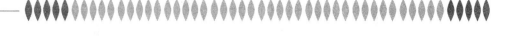

3. Prepare the grill or electric grilling machine for cooking.
4. If using a charcoal grill, oil the grid and place it over ashen coals or place the fish in a fish basket. Cook for 2 minutes, turn, and cook for about another 2 minutes, or until it is opaque in the center, and serve immediately.
5. If using an electric grilling machine, place the fish on a hot grill and cook for 1 to 1½ minutes, or until the fish is opaque in the center, and serve immediately.

Preparation time: *5 minutes*
Cooking time: *about 4 minutes on a grill; 1–1½ minutes in an electric grilling machine*
Makes 4 servings

Nutritional Breakdown (per serving)

Calories: 135	*Carbohydrates: 2 gm*	*Cholesterol: 36 mg*	*Saturated fat: 0 gm*
Protein: 24 gm	*Sodium: 63 mg*	*Fat: 3 gm*	*% calories fat: 19%*

Nutribite

Some health professionals recommend that we increase fish consumption to several servings a week, which may help lower the risk of heart disease. The fresher the fish, the more omega-3 fatty acids it contains; it's the omega-3s that are associated with maintaining clean arteries, platelets that don't get too sticky, normal cholesterol levels, and normal blood pressure.

Barbecued Monkfish with Butter-Wine Baste

Nicknamed "Monk" by my brothers and sisters, I answered to this name for years and passed it on to my second son, George. So I couldn't complete the fish section without including a recipe for monkfish. It's meaty, with a texture and sweet taste similar to lobster, another Foreman family favorite.

Butter-Wine Baste

¼ cup butter
2 garlic cloves, minced
⅓ cup dry white wine
¼ cup extra-virgin olive oil

3 tablespoons chopped fresh herbs, such as basil, thyme, chives, and parsley
2 teaspoons grated lemon zest

Monkfish

1–1½ pounds monkfish

Canola oil for the grid, if using a grill

1. To make the baste, melt 2 tablespoons of the butter in a small saucepan. Add the garlic and cook for 2 minutes. Stir in the white wine and cook until it is reduced to ¼ cup. Add the remaining butter and stir just until melted. Stir in the olive oil, herbs, and lemon zest. Set aside.
2. Brush the fish with the butter-wine mixture.
3. Prepare the grill or electric grilling machine.
4. If using a charcoal grill, oil the grid and place it 4 to 6 inches above ashen coals. Prick a piece of heavy aluminum foil several times with a fork and place the monkfish on it. Cook for 10 to 12 minutes, basting occasionally. When done, monkfish will be opaque in the center of the thickest part and firm to the touch.
5. If using an electric grilling machine, baste with the butter-wine mixture and place the fish on a hot grill. Cook for about 6 minutes, or until it is opaque in the center of the thickest part and firm to the touch. Baste about every 2 minutes with the butter-wine mixture.
6. Heat the remaining Butter-Wine Baste and serve on the side in small individual bowls for dipping as you would for lobster.

Preparation time: *5 minutes*
Cooking time: *about 15 minutes for the baste; 10–12 minutes on a grill; about 6 minutes in an electric grilling machine*
Makes 4 servings, 4–6 ounces each

Nutritional Breakdown (per serving)

Calories: 141	Carbohydrates: 1 gm	Cholesterol: 35 mg	Saturated fat: 2 gm
Protein: 16 gm	Sodium: 50 mg	Fat: 8 gm	% calories fat: 51%

George's Catfish Fillets with Sesame Crust

Catfish is my favorite, and I've heard it's also B. B. King's. Try it once and it may become yours, too. If you're using an outdoor grill, you will need to have a Griffo Grill (a special rack with small holes for grilling small foods and coated foods) to prevent the sesame seeds from falling off when you turn the fish. Or you may want to try the Cajun Spice Rub for Fish (page 38) for a blackened catfish grill.

Citrus Marinade

½ cup extra-virgin olive oil
½ cup white wine vinegar
1 tablespoon honey

2 teaspoons freshly grated lemon zest
Juice of ½ lemon
2 garlic cloves, minced

Catfish fillets

1½ pounds catfish fillets
¼ cup sesame seeds

Canola oil for the Griffo Grill, if using a grill

1. To make the marinade, combine all the ingredients in a medium bowl and stir well.
2. Wash the catfish fillets and pat dry. Add the catfish to the marinade, turning several times to coat well. Cover and refrigerate for 2 to 6 hours. Let sit at room temperature for 30 minutes before grilling. Drain from marinade and coat both sides of the fish with sesame seeds.

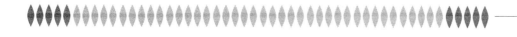
3. Prepare the grill or electric grilling machine for cooking.

4. If using a charcoal grill, place the grid above ashen coals. Oil the Griffo Grill and place the fish on top. Cook for about 4 minutes per side, or until whitish in the center.

5. If using an electric grilling machine, place the fish on a hot grill and cook for 4 to 5 minutes, or until whitish in the center. Usually fillets are quite a bit thicker at one end and need to be cut in half, with the different thicknesses grilled separately for more even cooking.

Preparation time: *5 minutes*
Cooking time: *about 8 minutes on a grill; 4–5 minutes in an electric grilling machine*
Makes 4 servings

Nutritional Breakdown (per serving)

Calories: 368	*Carbohydrates: 6 gm*	*Cholesterol: 55 mg*	*Saturated fat: 3 gm*
Protein: 37 gm	*Sodium: 94 mg*	*Fat: 22 gm*	*% calories fat: 54%*

Zesty Citrus-Thyme Shrimp Kabobs ♡

The Zesty Citrus-Thyme Marinade really makes this recipe. The kabobs go nicely over a bed of rice—brown basmati and wild rice would be a good blend. Heat the remaining marinade and drizzle on top of the kabobs before serving to flavor the rice as well.

Zesty Citrus-Thyme Marinade

Juice of 1 orange
2 tablespoons raspberry or red wine vinegar
2 tablespoons extra-virgin olive oil
1 tablespoon dried thyme

1 tablespoon minced garlic
1 teaspoon grated orange zest
½ teaspoon freshly ground black pepper

Shrimp Kabobs

1 pound shrimp (24–32 count), peeled and deveined

6 bamboo skewers, soaked in water for 15–30 minutes

Canola oil for the grid, if using a grill

1. To make the marinade, combine all the ingredients in a medium bowl and mix well.
2. Add the shrimp to the marinade, making sure all the shrimp are coated well. Cover and marinate for 1 to 2 hours in the refrigerator. Reserve the marinade and heat.
3. Thread the shrimp onto skewers (about 6 per skewer), allowing a little space in between each so they can cook evenly. (If using an electric grilling machine, cut the skewers to fit the machine.)
4. Prepare the grill or electric grilling machine for cooking.
5. If using a charcoal grill, oil the grid and place it over ashen coals. Place the skewers over direct heat and cook for 2 minutes. Turn and brush with marinade. Grill for 2 minutes longer, or just until the shrimp turn slightly pinkish in color (sometimes opaque white) and are just firm to the touch. Be careful not to overcook, as shrimp will become tough. (Larger shrimp may take a bit longer to cook.)
6. If using an electric grilling machine, place the skewers on a hot grill, drizzle a bit of the marinade over the top, cover, and cook for 1 minute and 10 to 15 seconds, or just until the shrimp turn slightly pinkish in color (sometimes opaque white) and are just firm to the touch. Be careful not to overcook, as shrimp will become tough. (Larger shrimp may take a few seconds longer to cook.)
7. To serve, place a skewer on each plate over a bed of rice. Drizzle a bit of the hot marinade over the top and serve immediately.

Preparation time: *10 minutes*
Cooking time: *4 minutes on a grill; 1 minute and 10–15 seconds in an electric grilling machine*
Makes 6 servings

Nutritional Breakdown (per serving)

Calories: 80	Carbohydrates: 2 gm	Cholesterol: 116 mg	Saturated fat: 0 gm
Protein: 13 gm	Sodium: 133 mg	Fat: 2 gm	% calories fat: 27%

Sea Scallop Brochettes with Tomato-Yogurt Sauce ♡

Brochette is the French word for skewer. These make a great late-summer or early-fall grill when tomatoes are vine-ripened and plentiful.

Tomato-Yogurt Sauce

1/2 cup minced onion

1/2 cup chopped, peeled, seeded fresh tomato

1/2 cup plain nonfat yogurt

1 tablespoon balsamic vinegar

2 tablespoons chopped fresh basil

1/4 teaspoon salt (optional)

1/4 teaspoon freshly ground black pepper

Scallop Brochettes

1 1/2 pounds large sea scallops, washed and
   patted dry

16 cherry tomatoes

8 bamboo skewers, soaked in water for
   15–30 minutes

2–3 tablespoons extra-virgin olive oil

1/2 teaspoon dried oregano

Canola oil for the grid, if using a grill

1. To make the Tomato-Yogurt Sauce, place all the ingredients in the bowl of a food processor or blender with a steel blade and process for about 1 minute. Pour the mixture into a small bowl, cover, and refrigerate until needed.

2. Thread the scallops onto skewers through the widest part, so they lie flat for more even cooking, and alternate them with cherry tomatoes. (If using an electric grilling machine, cut the skewers to fit the machine.) In a small bowl, mix the olive oil and oregano and brush the kabobs.

3. Prepare the grill or electric grilling machine for cooking.

4. If using a charcoal grill, oil the grid and place it above ashen coals. Place the scallop kabobs on the grill and cook for about 5 to 6 minutes, turning every 2 minutes and basting with the herbed oil. When done, the scallops will be white in the center and slightly firm to the touch. Be careful not to overcook or they will become dry and tough.

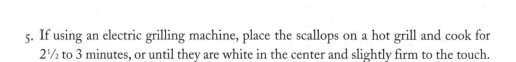
5. If using an electric grilling machine, place the scallops on a hot grill and cook for 2½ to 3 minutes, or until they are white in the center and slightly firm to the touch. Be careful not to overcook scallops, as they will be dry and tough.

6. To serve, place 2 scallop brochettes on each plate and serve with a dollop of Tomato-Yogurt Sauce on the side.

Preparation time: *10 minutes*
Cooking time: *about 5–6 minutes on a grill; about 3 minutes in an electric grilling machine.*
Makes 4 servings (2 brochettes each)

Nutritional Breakdown (per serving)

Calories: 219	*Carbohydrates: 13 gm*	*Cholesterol: 73 mg*	*Saturated fat: 0 gm*
Protein: 35 gm	*Sodium: 579 mg*	*Fat: 4 gm*	*% calories fat: 16%*

Thai Shrimp Kabobs

Cherie lived for a decade in Seattle, which has many Thai restaurants and markets, so Thai cooking is one of her favorite cuisines. Thai curry paste adds great flavor to a variety of dishes, and it comes in green, red, and yellow varieties. It can be found in the ethnic section of many grocery stores, Asian markets, and specialty food shops. Be sure to choose Thai curry paste rather than Indian curry paste for this recipe; the flavors are very different.

Thai Marinade

$1/4$ cup extra-virgin olive oil
$1/4$ cup raspberry vinegar
1 tablespoon honey
1 tablespoon minced garlic

1 tablespoon minced ginger
1–2 teaspoons Thai curry paste
$1/4$ teaspoon freshly ground black pepper

Shrimp Kabobs

16–20 jumbo shrimp (prawns), peeled and
   deveined
4 bamboo skewers, soaked in water for
   15–30 minutes, if using a grill

Canola oil for the grid, if using a grill
4 servings hot rice, such as jasmine or sweet
   brown rice

1. To make the marinade, combine all the ingredients in a medium bowl and mix well.
2. Add the shrimp and make sure all are covered with the marinade. Cover and marinate in the refrigerator for 2 to 4 hours. Let stand at room temperature for 30 minutes before grilling.
3. Thread the shrimp on skewers (about 4 per skewer) if using a grill, allowing a little space between each so they can cook evenly.
4. Prepare the grill or electric grilling machine for cooking.
5. If using a charcoal grill, set the skewers on an oiled grid over ashen coals and cook for 3 minutes. Turn, brush with marinade, and cook for about 2 more minutes, or just until the shrimp turn pinkish (sometimes opaque white) and just firm to the touch. Be careful not to overcook as the shrimp will become tough and rubbery.
6. If using an electric grilling machine, place the shrimp on a hot grill. Drizzle a bit of marinade over the top, cover, and cook for about 2 to $2^{1}/_{2}$ minutes, or just until the

shrimp turn pink (sometimes opaque white). Be careful not to overcook or the shrimp will become tough and rubbery.

7. Place 1 kabob or 4 to 5 prawns over hot rice on each plate. You can heat the remaining marinade and serve it on the side.

Preparation time: *10 minutes*
Cooking time: *about 5 minutes on a grill; 2–2½ minutes in an electric grilling machine*
Makes 4 servings

Nutritional Breakdown (per serving; does not include rice)

Calories: 158	*Carbohydrates: 3 gm*	*Cholesterol: 174 mg*	*Saturated fat: 1 gm*
Protein: 19 gm	*Sodium: 200 mg*	*Fat: 8 gm*	*% calories fat: 44%*

Nutribite

Known for its chili-rich curry paste, Thai cooking uses chilies in a variety of dishes and sauces. That's a healthy choice because, gram for gram, chili peppers contain more than seven times the vitamin C found in orange juice.

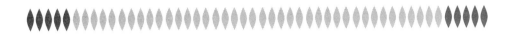

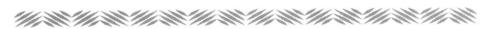

CHAPTER TEN

LAMB

LAMB IS A GOOD CHOICE FOR TODAY'S LIGHTER EATING, SINCE smaller amounts of lamb are considered standard fare. One or two 3-ounce loin chops are usually served per person. Lamb cooks quickly, is good in salads and kabobs, and since it is naturally tender, it is particularly suitable for grilling.

Grilling is an excellent way to cook lamb, since the excess fat, which can have an unpleasant taste, drips off. Chunks of meat from the shoulder or leg are good for kabobs, and are best if marinated first. Rib and lamb chops are the most popular cuts for grilling.

Lamb is a good source of protein, B vitamins, zinc, and chromium. Though not as low in fat as fish, seafood, or poultry, some cuts of lamb, such as those from the leg or shoulder, are lower in fat. Trimming away all visible fat from the meat before cooking reduces the fat content, in some cases by half.

Lamb may be a healthier animal protein choice over other red meat. Sheep are generally not raised under the same adverse conditions as many other livestock. Many are range-raised and are allowed to roam in pastures and graze at will. When that is the case, there usually is no need to give them large amounts of antibiotics. To make sure you're getting the healthiest meat, however, look for lamb that is labeled *grown naturally*—without hormones, steroids, growth stimulants, antibiotics, or other drugs.

TIPS FOR GRILLING LAMB

1. Lean cuts of lamb, such as the center cut from the leg, have little inside fat and should cook at a low temperature.

2. For low-temperature cooking, sear the meat for about 2 minutes per side on the hottest part of the grill and then move the meat to the cooler part for the remainder of cooking.

3. Lamb tastes best served while still slightly pink in the center. To test for doneness, press the meat with your fingers. Rare lamb does not resist; medium rare resists slightly; well done is firm to the touch.

4. Rib and loin chops are the most popular cuts for grilling. Shoulder chops are good if marinated first.

5. For flavorful, tender kabobs, use chunks of meat from the leg or shoulder and marinate them for 4 hours to overnight.

6. For food safety, always heat the marinade that the raw meat was sitting in before serving, and always wash the plate you carried raw meat on in hot, soapy water before using it again.

Grilled Lamb Salad
with Hot Minted-Wine Dressing

This is a delicious, light summer salad that makes a nice main-course dish. Serve it with warm pita bread and hummus dip for real Mideastern flavor. Hummus is a chick-pea–tahini spread that can be purchased at many grocery stores, health food stores, and Mideastern markets. It's also very easy to prepare at home and makes an excellent dip with warm pita bread.

Mint Marinade

¼ cup light soy sauce or tamari
1 tablespoon raspberry vinegar
1 tablespoon extra-virgin olive oil

1 tablespoon chopped fresh mint
¼ teaspoon freshly ground black pepper
Juice of ½ orange

Hot Minted-Wine Dressing

⅓ cup extra-virgin olive oil
¼ cup balsamic vinegar
¼ cup red wine
1 tablespoon Dijon mustard

3 teaspoons honey
¼ teaspoon freshly ground black pepper
1 garlic clove, minced
1 tablespoon chopped fresh mint

Grilled Lamb Salad

1½ pounds lamb top round cut into steaks, pounded and sliced against the grain*
Canola oil for the grid, if using a grill
4 bamboo skewers soaked in water for 15–30 minutes, if using a grill

2 cups romaine, washed, dried, and torn in bite-size pieces
2 cups red leaf lettuce or baby field greens
½ cup chopped green onions
10 cherry tomatoes, halved or quartered
¼ cup toasted pine nuts (optional)**

Garnish

4 sprigs fresh mint

* To help slice meat more thinly, place it in the freezer for 20 to 30 minutes first. If you want easy-to-chew meat, always slice it against the grain.
** To toast the nuts, place them on a baking sheet with a raised edge, and toast at 250° F for 25 to 30 minutes, or until they are golden. Be careful not to burn them. Remove the nuts from the oven and set aside to cool; they will become crunchier and more flavorful as they cool.

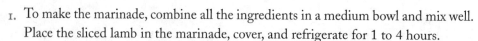

1. To make the marinade, combine all the ingredients in a medium bowl and mix well. Place the sliced lamb in the marinade, cover, and refrigerate for 1 to 4 hours.

2. To make the dressing, in a small saucepan, combine the olive oil, vinegar, wine, mustard, honey, pepper, and garlic. Whisk until mixed well. Heat over medium-low heat just until warm, and whisk occasionally to keep well blended. Remove from the heat and whisk in the mint. Reheat if needed and serve warm.

3. Prepare the grill or electric grilling machine for cooking.

4. If using a charcoal grill, thread the lamb onto skewers. Oil the grid and place it above ashen coals. Place the lamb skewers on the grid and cook for 2 minutes, baste, and turn. Cook for another 2 minutes for medium rare.

5. If using an electric grilling machine, place the lamb strips on a hot grill. Drizzle a bit of marinade over the top, and cook for 1 minute and 15 seconds for medium rare.

6. To assemble the salad, in a large salad bowl, combine the leafy greens, green onions, and tomatoes; toss to mix. Divide evenly among 4 plates. Top each salad with grilled lamb strips and spoon hot dressing over top. Sprinkle with toasted pine nuts, if using, and garnish with a sprig of mint. Serve immediately.

Preparation time: *about 20 minutes*

Cooking time: *3–4 minutes for the dressing; about 4 minutes on a grill; 1 minute and 15 seconds in an electric grilling machine*

Makes 4 servings

Nutritional Breakdown (per serving)

Calories: 539	*Carbohydrates: 12 gm*	*Cholesterol: 113 mg*	*Saturated fat: 9 gm*
Protein: 41 gm	*Sodium: 556 mg*	*Fat: 35 gm*	*% calories fat: 59%*

Nutribite

Dark leafy greens are excellent sources of beta-carotene, which research has shown is a prizewinning fighter in preventing cancer. There is no vitamin A in vegetables or fruit. It occurs as pro-vitamin A (beta-carotene and other carotenoids) and must be converted to active vitamin A by the body. The efficiency of conversion varies among individuals; however, beta-carotene is converted more efficiently than other carotenoids. Green and deep yellow-orange vegetables as well as deep yellow-orange fruits are the highest in beta-carotene.

Shish Kabobs with Fresh Mint Marinade

Shish kabob is an Arabic term meaning "skewered meat." The Fresh Mint marinade is ideal for lamb; it is delicious heated and drizzled over the kabobs and brown rice just before serving. Save a few extra sprigs of mint to make some refreshing minted iced water or iced tea to accompany your meal.

Fresh Mint Marinade

1/4 cup extra-virgin olive oil
1/4 cup red wine vinegar
1/4 cup minced onion
1/4 cup chopped fresh mint

2 tablespoons fresh lemon juice
3 garlic cloves, minced
1/4 teaspoon freshly ground black pepper

Shish Kabobs

2 pounds leg of lamb, trimmed of all fat
4 medium onions, cut into 16 wedges
16 pieces green pepper (cut them in squares)
16 cherry tomatoes

16 mushrooms, stemmed and washed
8 bamboo skewers, soaked in water for
    15–30 minutes, if using a grill
Canola oil for the grid, if using a grill

1. To prepare the marinade, place all the ingredients in a medium bowl, mix well, and set aside.
2. Cut the lamb into 1 1/2- to 2-inch chunks.
3. Blanch the onions and green peppers for 5 to 6 minutes, since they take longer to cook.
4. Divide the kabob ingredients into 8 portions and thread the skewers, alternating lamb, onion, green pepper, tomatoes, and mushrooms. (If using an electric grilling machine, cut the skewers to fit the machine.) Arrange the skewers in a shallow dish. Pour the marinade over the kabobs, cover, and refrigerate for 4 hours to overnight, turning occasionally. When ready to grill, remove the shish kabobs, and reserve the remaining marinade for basting. (It can also be heated and drizzled over the kabobs.) Let sit at room temperature 30 minutes before grilling.
5. Prepare the grill or electric grilling machine for cooking.
6. If using a charcoal grill, oil the grid and place the kabobs over ashen coals. Baste with some of the reserved marinade. Grill for about 7 minutes for medium doneness, turning and basting occasionally.

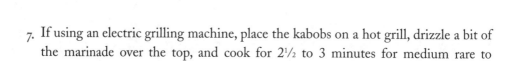

7. If using an electric grilling machine, place the kabobs on a hot grill, drizzle a bit of the marinade over the top, and cook for 2½ to 3 minutes for medium rare to medium doneness.

8. Serve the kabobs over a bed of brown rice or couscous, and drizzle a bit of the heated marinade over the top.

Preparation time: *10 minutes*
Cooking time: *5–6 minutes for the onions; 7 minutes on a grill; 2½–3 minutes in an electric grilling machine*
Makes 4 servings

Nutritional Breakdown (per serving)

Calories: 473	*Carbohydrates: 37 gm*	*Cholesterol: 115 mg*	*Saturated fat: 4 gm*
Protein: 42 gm	*Sodium: 261 mg*	*Fat: 17 gm*	*% calories fat: 33%*

Nutribite ≋

Mint has been used traditionally as an antibacterial and antiparasitic herb. It has also shown antispasmodic effects on smooth muscles such as the digestive system, and it is an effective digestive aid. Cooling to the palate, refreshing on a hot summer day, fresh mint is a nice addition to marinades and rubs for lamb, makes refreshing iced water or tea, and is good sprinkled on split pea soup, carrots, and zucchini.

George Foreman's Knock-Out-the-Fat Barbecue and Grilling Cookbook

Lamb Chops with Minted Tomato Salsa

Grilled lamb chops are flavorful by themselves, but when served with the Minted Tomato Salsa, we think you'll agree, they are outstanding! Couscous and grilled zucchini make a nice accompaniment for a special dinner presentation. Spoon a bit of the salsa over the couscous for added flavor.

Balsamic-Mint Marinade

¼ cup balsamic vinegar

2 tablespoons chopped fresh mint leaves or 1 tablespoon dried

1 garlic clove, minced

½ teaspoon freshly ground black pepper

Salt to taste (optional)

Grilled Lamb Chops

8 loin or rib lamb chops, about 1½ inches thick, trimmed of excess fat

Canola oil for the grid, if using a grill

Minted Tomato Salsa

2 medium tomatoes, peeled, seeded, and chopped

2 green onions, chopped

2 garlic cloves, finely minced

4 tablespoons tomato paste

2 tablespoons chopped mild green chilies

2 tablespoons chopped fresh mint leaves, or 1 tablespoon dried

1 tablespoon fresh lime juice

1 tablespoon extra-virgin olive oil

½ teaspoon lemon zest

½ teaspoon dried rosemary

Salt and pepper to taste (optional)

1. To make the marinade, combine all the ingredients in a large, shallow bowl.
2. Add the lamb chops to the marinade, cover, and marinate for 4 hours to overnight in the refrigerator. Remove from refrigerator and let sit at room temperature for 30 minutes before grilling.
3. To make the salsa, combine all the ingredients in a medium bowl and mix well. Cover and chill until ready to serve.
4. Prepare the grill or electric grilling machine for cooking.
5. If using a charcoal grill, place the chops on an oiled grid over ashen coals and grill for 2 to 3 minutes, turn, and grill for another 2 to 3 minutes for medium rare and 7

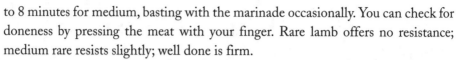
to 8 minutes for medium, basting with the marinade occasionally. You can check for doneness by pressing the meat with your finger. Rare lamb offers no resistance; medium rare resists slightly; well done is firm.

6. If using an electric grilling machine, place the lamb chops on a hot grill, drizzle a bit of the marinade over the chops, and grill for about 5 minutes for medium rare or about 5½ minutes for medium doneness. You can check for doneness by pressing the meat with your finger. Rare lamb offers no resistance; medium rare resists slightly; well done is firm.

7. Place 2 lamb chops on each plate and spoon a bit of salsa on top of each. Serve the remaining salsa on the side.

Preparation time: *20 minutes*
Cooking time: *6 minutes on a grill; 5 minutes in an electric grilling machine*
Makes 4 servings

Nutritional Breakdown (per serving)

Calories: 413	*Carbohydrates: 9 gm*	*Cholesterol: 148 mg*	*Saturated fat: 7 gm*
Protein: 47 gm	*Sodium: 276 mg*	*Fat: 20 mg*	*% calories fat: 45%*

Nutribite

All around the world, in surveys of people who are cancer-free, the tomato has appeared on many people's lists of foods they frequently eat. It is distinguished for its particular carotene—lycopene. Over 600 carotenes have been identified, and scientists have found that many of them help prevent cancer.

Joan's Rosemary Lamb Chops

One of the most memorable meals I ever had was a dinner my wife made just for me—lamb and potatoes. Shortly after Joan and I were married, I started teaching her how to cook my favorite foods and dishes like my mother made. Then one day I came home to lamb and potatoes on the grill—Joan's own idea–and our own family tradition began. These lamb chops taste great served with Roasted New Potatoes with Garlic and Rosemary (page 158).

Rosemary Marinade

¼ cup extra-virgin olive oil

¼ cup balsamic vinegar

2 tablespoons chopped fresh rosemary, stemmed, or 1 tablespoon dried

1 tablespoon fresh lime juice

¼ teaspoon freshly ground black pepper

2 garlic cloves, minced

1 green onion, chopped

Grilled Lamb Chops

8 loin lamb chops

Canola oil for the grid, if using a grill

1. To make the marinade, combine all the ingredients in a medium shallow bowl and mix well.
2. Add the lamb chops to the marinade and make sure they are completely coated with the mixture. Cover and place them in the refrigerator to marinate for 4 hours to overnight. Bring to room temperature 30 minutes before grilling.
3. Prepare the grill or electric grilling machine for cooking.
4. If using a charcoal grill, place the chops on an oiled grid above ashen coals and grill for about 6 minutes per side for medium rare. Brush with marinade before turning.
5. If using an electric grilling machine, place the lamb chops on a hot grill, drizzle a bit of marinade over the top, and cook for 4 to 6 minutes for medium rare.

Preparation time: *5 minutes*
Cooking time: *about 12 minutes on a grill; 5–6 minutes in an electric grilling machine*
Makes 4 servings (2 chops each)

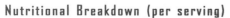

Nutritional Breakdown (per serving)

Calories: 412	Carbohydrates: 2 gm	Cholesterol: 148 mg	Saturated fat: 7 gm
Protein: 45 gm	Sodium: 113 mg	Fat: 23 gm	% calories fat: 52%

Nutribite ≋

Rosemary has been used for centuries to aid digestion. It is also known to improve circulation and strengthen fragile blood vessels due to the effect of a particular flavonoid known as diosmin.

Spice-and-Herb-Crusted Lamb with Yogurt Sauce

≋ The crust is hot and spicy; the yogurt sauce is cooling. It's the right blend of flavors for creating your own memorable meal.

Spice-and-Herb-Crusted Lamb

4 tablespoons Spice and Herb Rub for
　Lamb (page 41)
8 shoulder lamb chops, trimmed of fat,
　1/4 inch thick

Canola oil for brushing the lamb and the
　grid, if using a grill

Yogurt Sauce

1/3 cup plain nonfat yogurt
2 tablespoons fresh lemon juice
1 teaspoon grated ginger
3 garlic cloves, minced
2 green onions, chopped
1 teaspoon ground cumin

1/4 teaspoon ground turmeric
1/4 teaspoon ground cloves
1/4 teaspoon freshly ground black pepper
1/4 teaspoon salt
1/8 teaspoon ground cardamom (optional)

Garnish

8 sprigs cilantro

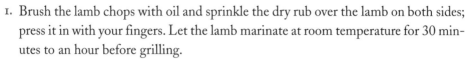
1. Brush the lamb chops with oil and sprinkle the dry rub over the lamb on both sides; press it in with your fingers. Let the lamb marinate at room temperature for 30 minutes to an hour before grilling.

2. To prepare the Yogurt Sauce, spoon the yogurt into a small bowl. Stir in the lemon juice, ginger, garlic, and green onions. Mix in the cumin, turmeric, cloves, pepper, salt, and cardamom, if using, until well blended. Cover and refrigerate until needed.

3. Prepare the grill or electric grilling machine for cooking.

4. If using a charcoal grill, oil the grid and place it above ashen coals. Place the lamb over direct heat and grill for about 6 minutes per side for medium rare. Check for doneness by pressing the meat with your fingertips. Rare lamb offers no resistance; medium rare resists slightly; well done is firm.

5. If using an electric grilling machine, place the lamb on a hot grill and cook for 4 to 6 minutes for medium rare. Check for doneness by pressing the meat with your fingertips. Rare lamb offers no resistance; medium rare resists slightly; well done is firm.

6. To serve, place the lamb chops on individual plates with a dollop of Yogurt Sauce and garnish with sprigs of cilantro.

Preparation time: *10 minutes*
Cooking time: *about 12 minutes on a grill; 4–6 minutes in an electric grilling machine*
Makes 4 servings

Nutritional Breakdown (per serving)

Calories: 414	*Carbohydrates: 3 gm*	*Cholesterol: 148 mg*	*Saturated fat: 8 gm*
Protein: 45 gm	*Sodium: 289 mg*	*Fat: 23 gm*	*% calories fat: 51%*

Grilled Lamb Chops with Plum Sauce

〰 Cherie's husband loves lamb, but red meat is something she makes only on special occasions. Since John was one of the taste-testers for this cookbook, sampling the lamb recipes was a treat, to say the least. He gave two thumbs up for our Plum Sauce! We suggest serving it with couscous and summer squash.

Lamb Chops

8 lamb loin chops, 1 inch thick, trimmed of all visible fat

Canola oil for brushing the lamb and the grid, if using a grill

Plum Sauce

3 large or 4 medium ripe purple or blue plums, fresh or canned, pitted and sliced

½ cup grape juice, freshly made or bottled

2 tablespoons chopped fresh rosemary, stemmed, or 1 tablespoon dried

1 tablespoon honey

1 tablespoon cornstarch

2 tablespoons water

To prepare the lamb chops:

1. Prepare the grill or electric grilling machine.
2. If using a charcoal grill, oil the grid and place it above ashen coals. Brush the chops on both sides with oil and place them directly over the heat. Grill for 6 minutes per side for medium rare. You can check for doneness by pressing the meat with your fingertips. Rare lamb offers no resistance; medium rare resists slightly; well done is firm.
3. If using an electric grilling machine, place the chops on a hot grill (no need for oil) and cook for about 4 to 6 minutes for medium rare. You can check for doneness by pressing the meat with your fingertips. Rare lamb offers no resistance; medium rare resists slightly; well done is firm.

To make the sauce:

1. While the lamb chops are cooking, in a medium saucepan combine the plums, grape juice, rosemary, and honey. Bring to a boil; reduce the heat, cover, and simmer for 3 minutes if the plums are canned or for 6 to 8 minutes if the plums are fresh.

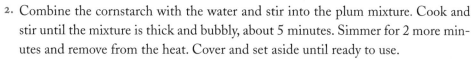

2. Combine the cornstarch with the water and stir into the plum mixture. Cook and stir until the mixture is thick and bubbly, about 5 minutes. Simmer for 2 more minutes and remove from the heat. Cover and set aside until ready to use.

3. Serve the lamb chops with hot Plum Sauce on the side.

Preparation time: *10 minutes*

Cooking time: *10–15 minutes for the Plum Sauce; about 12 minutes for lamb chops on a grill;*
4–6 minutes for lamb chops in an electric grilling machine

Makes 4 servings

Nutritional Breakdown (per serving)

Calories: 396	*Carbohydrates: 13 gm*	*Cholesterol: 148 mg*	*Saturated fat: 6 gm*
Protein: 46 gm	*Sodium: 113 mg*	*Fat: 17 gm*	*% calories fat: 39%*

POULTRY

ONE OF AMERICA'S MOST POPULAR FOODS AT PICNICS AND BACK-
yard parties, barbecued chicken is a tradition that's here to stay. Chicken is versatile and
easy to barbecue, and it absorbs the flavors of most sauces very well. The key to good
barbecue is cooking the chicken slowly over a drip pan with indirect heat.

Chicken is also ideal for grilling because it takes on the flavors of marinades
readily, and it is excellent in kabobs. We used skinless chicken in our grilling, and it
turned out moist and juicy every time. Just watch it closely, baste it often, and turn it
frequently.

Chicken, turkey, and other poultry products provide protein and B vitamins.
Turkey is rich in the amino acid tryptophan, which helps promote restful sleep. (No
wonder we often feel like taking a nap after Thanksgiving dinner!)

To keep the fat content as low as possible, remove the skin from chicken or
turkey before eating and preferably before cooking. To keep your dishes low in fat, cook
poultry without added fat whenever possible. For the healthiest poultry, buy the fresh-
est birds available. And look for labels that say *naturally grown*—meaning the poultry
was grown without hormones, growth stimulants, antibiotics, steroids, or any other
drugs. *Naturally grown* should also mean that the birds have been raised free of the
confinement of small cages, and kept in pens or loose, where they could hunt and peck
for their food. These practices result in healthier birds, which produce healthier food.
If your market doesn't carry naturally grown poultry products, ask for them or order
them yourself by mail.

TIPS FOR GRILLING AND BARBECUING POULTRY

1. When buying chicken, look for relatively dry skin and an even color. Avoid chicken with excess liquid in the package, torn wrapping, or off-coloration. There should be no unpleasant odor and no stickiness when touched.

2. *Salmonella* bacteria is found in chicken, which can cause food poisoning in humans and other warm-blooded animals. See pages 23–24 for safe handling tips.

3. Chicken is done when it reaches a temperature of 165°F. The meat should be white and the juices should run clear.

4. Marinating chicken overnight is not recommended, since it can become too tender and fall apart on the grill. Remember to always heat marinade used for raw poultry well before serving as a sauce.

5. To grill chicken, place it on the hottest part of the grill and sear it for 3 minutes on each side. Then move it to a slightly cooler area and baste it often, turning it frequently until done.

6. To barbecue chicken, place it over a drip pan and cook it slowly over indirect heat. Baste it with a tomato-based sauce when it's half done, since this type of sauce tends to burn.

7. Remember: Always wash the platter on which you carried raw poultry to the grill in hot, soapy water before you use it for any other food.

Ranch-Style Honey Barbecued Chicken

Though barbecue sauce for chicken should be a bit sweeter than sauce for beef or pork, it does not need to be made with refined sugars to be delicious. We think our sauce, made with honey and a touch of molasses, is better than *any* sugar-laced version. But then you'll have to judge for yourself. The sauce will keep for several weeks in the refrigerator or it can be frozen. If it is frozen, add 2 to 4 tablespoons of water to reconstitute it.

Honey Barbecue Sauce

2 tablespoons extra-virgin olive oil

½ cup minced onion

½ cup minced celery

½ cup minced green bell pepper

1 (10 ¾ ounce) can tomato puree

½ cup chicken broth

¾ cup honey

1 tablespoon blackstrap molasses

¼ cup apple cider vinegar

1 tablespoon Dijon mustard

1 tablespoon chili powder

2 garlic cloves, minced

2 bay leaves

Barbecued Chicken

1 (2½ to 3 pound) chicken, cut up (4 bone-less, skinless chicken breasts work best in an electric grilling machine)

Canola oil for the grid, if using a grill

To make the barbecue sauce:

1. Add the olive oil and vegetables to a medium saucepan, and cook over medium-high heat for about 10 minutes, or until the vegetables are soft.
2. Add the tomato puree and chicken broth, and cook for another 2 minutes.
3. Stir in the honey and molasses, mixing well. Then add the apple cider vinegar, mustard, chili powder, garlic, and bay leaves, and simmer for 1 hour. Serve warm as a finishing and table sauce. (Remove the bay leaves before serving.)

To barbecue the chicken:

1. Prepare the grill or electric grilling machine for cooking.
2. If using a charcoal grill, oil the grid and place it over ashen coals. Place the chicken directly over the heat and lightly brown it on both sides, allowing about 3 minutes

per side. Then move the chicken over a drip pan and close the lid. After 15 minutes turn the chicken and baste with barbecue sauce. After another 15 minutes, place a piece of heavy-duty aluminum foil that has been pricked with a fork in several places under the chicken. Baste the chicken with barbecue sauce and close the lid. Every 10 minutes baste the chicken with sauce and turn it over. The chicken should be done in 45 minutes to an hour. Heat the remaining sauce and serve on the side.

3. If using an electric grilling machine, spread barbecue sauce over boneless, skinless chicken breasts and place them on a hot grill. Cook for 2 to 2½ minutes, or until no pink meat remains. Heat the remaining sauce and serve on the side.

Preparation time: *10 minutes*
Cooking time: *1 hour and 10 minutes for the sauce; 45 minutes–1 hour on a grill; 2–2½ minutes in an electric grilling machine for boneless chicken breasts*
Makes 4 servings

Nutritional Breakdown (per serving)

Calories: 764	*Carbohydrates: 68 gm*	*Cholesterol: 175 mg*	*Saturated fat: 7 gm*
Protein: 58 gm	*Sodium: 692 mg*	*Fat: 29 gm*	*% calories fat: 34%*

Cherie's Barbecued Chicken with Apple-Cinnamon Sauce

In honor of Washington, the apple state, where Cherie spent a lot of years barbecuing, she's developed her own apple barbecue sauce. Both of us think it could take a prize. Its sweet, spicy flavor turns barbecued chicken into a gourmet feast. The Barbecued Sweet Potato–Apple Kabobs (page 156) would make a nice accompaniment.

Apple-Cinnamon Barbecue Sauce

1 tablespoon extra-virgin olive oil
1/4 cup minced onion
1/4 cup minced green bell pepper
2 garlic cloves, minced
1 (10 3/4 ounce) can tomato puree
1/4 cup apple cider
1/4 cup apple cider vinegar

1/4 cup honey
1/4 cup light soy sauce or tamari
2 tablespoons Worcestershire sauce
1 teaspoon ground cinnamon
1/2 sweet apple (preferably Golden Delicious), peeled and grated

Barbecued Chicken

1 (2 1/2 to 3 pound) chicken, cut up (4 boneless, skinless chicken breasts work best in an electric grilling machine)

Canola oil for the grid, if using a grill

To make the barbecue sauce:

1. Heat the oil in a medium saucepan over medium-high heat and add the onion, bell pepper, and garlic. Sauté for about 10 minutes, or until tender.
2. Add all the remaining ingredients and simmer for 30 minutes. Add the grated apple for the last 5 minutes. Set aside and reheat when ready to use as a finishing and table sauce.

To barbecue the chicken:

1. Prepare the grill or electric grilling machine for cooking.
2. If using a charcoal grill, oil the grid and place it above ashen coals. Place the chicken directly over the heat and lightly brown it on both sides, allowing about 3 minutes

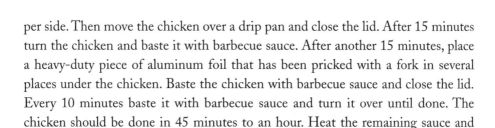

per side. Then move the chicken over a drip pan and close the lid. After 15 minutes turn the chicken and baste it with barbecue sauce. After another 15 minutes, place a heavy-duty piece of aluminum foil that has been pricked with a fork in several places under the chicken. Baste the chicken with barbecue sauce and close the lid. Every 10 minutes baste it with barbecue sauce and turn it over until done. The chicken should be done in 45 minutes to an hour. Heat the remaining sauce and serve on the side.

3. If using an electric grilling machine, spread barbecue sauce over both sides of the boneless chicken breasts. Grill for 2 to 2½ minutes, or until no pink meat remains. Heat the remaining sauce and serve on the side.

Preparation time: *10 minutes*

Cooking time: *40 minutes for the sauce; 45 minutes–1 hour on a grill; 2–2½ minutes in an electric grilling machine for boneless chicken breasts*

Makes 4 servings

Nutritional Breakdown (per serving)

Calories: 657	*Carbohydrates: 59 gm*	*Cholesterol: 175 mg*	*Saturated fat: 7 gm*
Protein: 59 gm	*Sodium: 1177 mg*	*Fat: 26 gm*	*% calories fat: 34%*

Nutribite

How many times have you heard someone recite the old adage "An apple a day keeps the doctor away"? If you've been tempted to think that's just a bit of folklore, think again—this time from a scientific point of view. Canadian researchers poured apple juice in test tubes and found it killed certain viruses. And U.S. researchers found that those who eat the most apples have fewer colds, flu, and upper respiratory infections, and less sickness in general.

Barbecued Chicken with Sweet Mustard Sauce

Barbecue sauces have wide regional variations, and which area has the best sauce is a topic that is hotly debated. South Carolina is known for its mustard-based sauces. Our mustard sauce has other regional influences, like fresh rosemary, which has always grown wild around the Mediterranean coasts. Today, with the popularity of fresh herbs, rosemary can be found in the produce section of many grocery stores. Cherie has found fresh rosemary even in small-town markets along northeastern Pennsylvania backroads.

Sweet Mustard Sauce

½ cup honey
¼ cup chicken broth
2 tablespoons Dijon mustard
2 tablespoons butter

2 tablespoons chopped fresh rosemary,
  stemmed, or 1 tablespoon dried
¼ teaspoon freshly ground black pepper

Barbecued Chicken

1 (2½ to 3 pound) chicken, cut up (4 bone-
  less, skinless chicken breasts work best in
  an electric grilling machine)

Canola oil for the grid, if using a grill

1. To make the Sweet Mustard Sauce, combine all the ingredients in a medium saucepan and cook over medium heat for 10 to 15 minutes, or until reduced by about one half. Reheat before using as a finishing and table sauce.
2. Prepare the grill or electric grilling machine for cooking.
3. If using a charcoal grill, oil the grid and place it above ashen coals. Put the chicken directly over the coals and sear it on both sides, allowing about 3 minutes per side. Then move the chicken over a drip pan and close the lid. After 15 minutes turn the chicken and baste with barbecue sauce. After another 15 minutes, place a piece of heavy-duty aluminum foil that has been pricked with holes under the chicken. Baste it with barbecue sauce and close the lid. Every 10 minutes baste the chicken with sauce and turn it over until done. The chicken should be done in 45 minutes to an hour. Heat the remaining sauce and serve on the side.

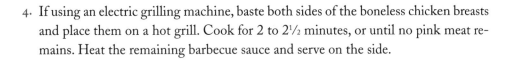

4. If using an electric grilling machine, baste both sides of the boneless chicken breasts and place them on a hot grill. Cook for 2 to 2½ minutes, or until no pink meat remains. Heat the remaining barbecue sauce and serve on the side.

Preparation time: *5 minutes*
Cooking time: *10–15 minutes for the sauce; 45 minutes–1 hour on a grill; 2–2½ minutes in an electric grilling machine for boneless chicken breasts*
Makes 4 servings

Nutrition Breakdown (per serving)

Calories: 628	*Carbohydrates: 35 gm*	*Cholesterol: 190 mg*	*Saturated fat: 10 gm*
Protein: 57 gm	*Sodium: 504 mg*	*Fat: 28 gm*	*% calories fat: 41%*

Nutribite 〰

Mustard is warming and stimulating to the digestive tract. As an herbal remedy, it has been used for coughs, colds, and indigestion.

Texas Cowboy BBQ Drumsticks ♡

〰 Are you ready for a finger-lickin' favorite? These drumsticks can be served as hors d'oeuvres or as a main course with all the backyard-party favorites like potato salad, garlic bread, and ice-cold watermelon.

1 recipe LBJ's Texas Barbecue Sauce (page 42) or your favorite sauce
Skinless chicken drumsticks for 4 (about 1¼ pounds)

Canola oil for the grid (because of the bones, drumsticks do not cook well in an electric grilling machine)

1. Prepare the grill for cooking.
2. Oil the grid and place it above ashen coals. Place the drumsticks directly over the heat and sear for about 3 minutes on each side. Then move them over a drip pan and close the lid. After 10 minutes, brush with barbecue sauce. Cook for about 3 min-

utes, turn the drumsticks over, and baste with sauce. Cook for another 3 minutes, or until done, turning and basting frequently. (When drumsticks are done, the juices should run clear and no pink remain.) Spoon warm barbecue sauce over the drumsticks and serve hot.

Preparation time: *about 5 minutes*
Cooking time: *about 22 minutes*
Makes 4 servings

Nutritional Breakdown (per serving)

Calories: 285	*Carbohydrates: 35 gm*	*Cholesterol: 55 mg*	*Saturated fat: 2 gm*
Protein: 19 gm	*Sodium: 812 mg*	*Fat: 9 gm*	*% calories fat: 26%*

For barbecued chicken that is juicy and not covered with black char, cook it slowly over indirect heat after searing over direct heat. Wait until it is halfway done before basting it with a tomato-based sauce. And place it on heavy aluminum foil that has been pricked with a few holes before turning the sauce-basted side toward the fire.

Grilled Chicken Parmesan

≈ Traditionally, chicken Parmesan is breaded and fried, making it a very high-fat food. Juicy and tender, this version is much lower in fat because the chicken is grilled, and it is fresher tasting, since we use fresh tomatoes rather than tomato sauce to top the chicken breasts. This dish goes well with a side of pasta and steamed vegetables.

Fresh Basil–Balsamic Vinegar Marinade

¼ cup extra-virgin olive oil
¼ cup balsamic vinegar
2 tablespoons chopped fresh basil or
    1 tablespoon dried (if using dried basil,
    add 2 teaspoons dried rosemary and
    2 teaspoons dried oregano)

1½ tablespoons minced garlic
1 tablespoon fresh lemon juice

Chicken Parmesan

4 skinless chicken breasts, deboned and flat-
    tened
4 ½-inch slices ripe tomato

¼ cup freshly grated Parmesan cheese
Canola oil for the grid, if using a grill

1. To make the marinade, combine all the ingredients in a medium bowl.
2. Pour the marinade over the chicken in a shallow bowl and marinate for 3 to 6 hours in the refrigerator. Let it sit at room temperature for 30 minutes before grilling. When ready to grill, drain the chicken from the marinade and reserve the remaining marinade for basting.
3. Prepare the grill or electric grilling machine for cooking.
4. If using a grill, place the chicken on an oiled grid directly over ashen coals and cover. Grill for 12 to 15 minutes, or until the chicken meat is completely white and the juices run clear. Be careful not to overcook the chicken or it will be tough. (Boneless chicken breasts need to be watched more closely and turned and basted often.) About 4 minutes before the chicken is done, place tomato slices on the outer edge of the grid and grill 2 minutes on each side. When the tomatoes are nicely grilled, top each chicken breast with a slice of tomato and about a tablespoon of grated

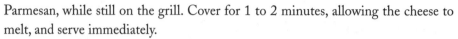

Parmesan, while still on the grill. Cover for 1 to 2 minutes, allowing the cheese to melt, and serve immediately.

5. If using an electric grilling machine, place the chicken breasts on a hot grill, drizzle a bit of the marinade over the top, and cook for about 2 minutes, or until the chicken is completely white and the juices run clear. Top each chicken breast with a slice of tomato, close the lid, and grill for 5 seconds. Then top each breast with about 1 tablespoon of grated Parmesan cheese, brush the upper grill with a little oil so the cheese won't stick, and close the lid for about 10 seconds so the cheese will melt. Serve immediately.

Preparation time: *10 minutes*
Cooking time: *about 15 minutes on a grill; about 2 minutes in an electric grilling machine*
Makes 4 servings

Nutritional Breakdown (per serving)

Calories: 385	*Carbohydrates: 3 gm*	*Cholesterol: 151 mg*	*Saturated fat: 4 gm*
Protein: 56 gm	*Sodium: 245 mg*	*Fat: 15 gm*	*% calories fat: 36%*

Boneless Chicken Breasts
with Fat-Free Garlic-Wine Marinade ♡

Our boneless, skinless chicken breasts taste flavorful and juicy when marinated in a garlic-wine marinade that's fat-free to boot! Top a plate of green salad with a grilled chicken breast, or serve one over brown rice or linguine for a quick and easy evening meal that's truly gourmet. For a busy weeknight supper, you can mix the marinade the day before and marinate the chicken in it for 2 to 6 hours. With just a little planning, dinner can be on the table in less than 30 minutes.

1 recipe Fat-Free Garlic-Wine Marinade   *Canola oil for the grid, if using a grill*
(page 34)
4 skinless chicken breasts, deboned and
flattened

1. Pour the marinade over the chicken in a shallow bowl and marinate for 2 to 6 hours. When ready to grill, drain the chicken and reserve the remaining marinade to baste the breasts as they grill.
2. Prepare the grill or electric grilling machine for cooking.
3. If using a charcoal grill, place the chicken breasts on an oiled grid directly over ashen coals and cover. Grill for 12 to 15 minutes, or until the chicken is completely white in the center and the juices run clear. Be careful not to overcook or it will be tough. (Boneless chicken breasts need to be watched more closely and basted and turned frequently.) Serve immediately.
4. If using an electric grilling machine, place the chicken breasts on a hot grill, drizzle a bit of the marinade over the top, and cook for about 2 minutes, or until the chicken is completely white in the center and the juices run clear. Serve immediately.

Preparation time: *5 minutes*
Cooking time: *12–15 minutes on a grill; about 2 minutes in an electric grilling machine*
Makes 4 servings

Nutritional Breakdown (per serving)

Calories: 297	*Carbohydrates: 2 gm*	*Cholesterol: 146 mg*	*Saturated fat: 2 gm*
Protein: 54 gm	*Sodium: 127 mg*	*Fat: 6 gm*	*% calories fat: 20%*

Stuffed Chicken Breasts with Peach-Pecan Stuffing

Sweet, crunchy pecan stuffing makes this chicken grill a treat any time, whether it's a special occasion or a relaxing family dinner. Testing this recipe in Cherie's kitchen was a treat for more than one reason. The dried peaches were sent as a sample from Gleanings for the Hungry, an organization that dries fruit and sends it to feed poor people in Manila who live off the dump. Perhaps the stuffing tasted exceptionally good to us because of all the love wrapped around the dried peaches.

Marinade

¼ cup extra-virgin olive oil

¼ cup raspberry vinegar

2 tablespoons fresh orange juice

1 tablespoon honey

2 teaspoons crushed sage

1 teaspoon dried oregano

¼ teaspoon freshly ground black pepper

2 garlic cloves, minced

Peach-Pecan Stuffing

2 tablespoons extra-virgin olive oil

½ cup chopped onion

½ cup chopped celery

2 garlic cloves, minced

3 cups bread stuffing or 4 slices toasted
whole-grain bread, cubed

½–¾ cup chicken broth

½ cup chopped dried peaches (dried apricots
can be substituted)

2 tablespoons crushed sage

1 tablespoon dried oregano

1 tablespoon chopped fresh parsley

½ cup chopped toasted pecans*

Grilled Chicken Breasts

4 chicken breasts, boned, skinned, and
halved

Wooden toothpicks for closing chicken breast
pockets

Canola oil for the grid, if using a grill

To make the marinade:

1. Combine all the marinade ingredients in a medium, shallow bowl, stirring to combine well.
2. With a small, sharp knife, make a deep, horizontal cut in each chicken breast. Add the chicken to the marinade, making sure the marinade coats the inside of the pocket. Cover, and refrigerate for 2 to 6 hours.

To make the stuffing:

1. In a medium saucepan over medium-high heat, add the oil, onion, celery, and garlic. Sauté for about 10 minutes, or until the vegetables are tender.
2. Reduce the heat to medium low and add the bread stuffing or cubed bread, ½ cup of the chicken broth, dried peaches, sage, oregano, and parsley. Stir to combine well.

*To toast nuts, place them whole (chop them after toasting) on a baking sheet with an edge, and toast at 250° F for 25 to 30 minutes, or until they are golden. Be careful not to burn them. Remove nuts from the oven and cool before chopping; they will become crunchier and more flavorful as they cool.

Add more chicken broth if the stuffing is too dry. Remove from the heat, stir in the toasted pecans, and set aside.

To grill the chicken:

1. Stuff each chicken breast with 2 to 3 tablespoons of stuffing and close each pocket with toothpicks to hold the stuffing inside.
2. Prepare the grill or electric grilling machine for cooking.
3. If using a charcoal grill, oil the grid and place it above ashen coals. Place the chicken breasts directly over the fire and sear, about 2 minutes on each side. Then move the chicken to a cooler part of the grill and cook over indirect heat for 4 to 6 minutes on each side, basting two or three times, or until the chicken meat is completely white and the juices run clear. Be careful not to overcook, as it will become dry and tough.
4. If using an electric grilling machine, place the chicken breasts on a hot grill, drizzle a bit of the marinade over the top, and cook for $3\frac{1}{2}$ to 4 minutes, or until the chicken meat is completely white and the juices run clear. Be careful not to overcook, as it will become dry and tough.

Preparation time: *15 minutes*
Cooking time: *about 12 minutes for the stuffing; 12–16 minutes on a grill; $3\frac{1}{2}$–4 minutes in an electric grilling machine*
Makes 4 servings

Nutritional Breakdown (per serving)

Calories: 592	*Carbohydrates: 20 gm*	*Cholesterol: 146 mg*	*Saturated fat: 5 gm*
Protein: 59 gm	*Sodium: 483 mg*	*Fat: 31 gm*	*% calories fat: 46%*

Chicken Kabobs with Peanut Dipping Sauce

Chicken kabobs make a great entrée or appetizer. Serve them over a bed of saffron or jasmine rice as a main dish, with peanut sauce on the side, or as an appetizer with peanut sauce while your entrée is grilling.

Marinade

¹⁄₄ cup light soy sauce or tamari
2 tablespoons honey
1 tablespoon rice vinegar
1 tablespoon peanut oil

1 tablespoon minced ginger
2 teaspoons minced garlic
1 teaspoon ground coriander

Chicken Kabobs

2 chicken breasts, boned, skinned, and cut in half
¹⁄₂ red bell pepper, cut into ¹⁄₂-inch cubes
8 green onions, green tops cut to 2 inches

Canola oil for the grid, if using a grill
8 bamboo skewers, soaked in water for 15–30 minutes; cut skewers in half for appetizers

Peanut Sauce

3 tablespoons peanut oil
1 cup chopped onion
¹⁄₄ cup minced ginger
2 garlic cloves, minced
1 cup crunchy or creamy peanut butter (preferably all-natural, only salt added)
³⁄₄ cup coconut milk

¹⁄₃ cup light soy sauce or tamari
¹⁄₄ cup honey
3 tablespoons fresh lime juice
2 teaspoons Thai curry paste (red, green, or yellow)
¹⁄₄ cup chopped cilantro leaves

To make the marinade:

1. Combine all the marinade ingredients in a medium bowl and mix well.
2. Cut each half-breast into 4 lengthwise strips, and then cut them in thirds. You should have bite-size chunks.

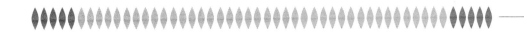
3. Add the chicken to the marinade, cover, and marinate in the refrigerator for 2–6 hours.

To make the peanut sauce:

1. In a medium saucepan over medium-high heat, add the oil, onion, ginger, and garlic. Sauté for about 10 minutes, or until the vegetables are tender.
2. Stir in the peanut butter, coconut milk, soy sauce, honey, lime juice, and curry paste. Reduce the heat to low and simmer for about 5 minutes, stirring occasionally.
3. Remove the pan from the heat and stir in the cilantro. Serve warm. If the mixture is too thick, thin it with coconut milk or water.
4. Unused sauce can be refrigerated up to a week.

To make the kabobs:

1. Parboil the bell pepper cubes for about 5 minutes.
2. Thread the chicken chunks onto skewers, with bell pepper cubes interspersed and 1 green onion in the middle of each skewer. (Omit the onions if making appetizers.)
3. Prepare the grill or electric grilling machine.
4. If using a charcoal grill, oil the grid and place it above ashen coals. Grill kabobs over direct heat for 5 to 6 minutes, or until the chicken meat is completely white and the juices run clear, turning once and basting before turning. Serve with Peanut Sauce on the side.
5. If using an electric grilling machine, place the kabobs on a hot grill, drizzle a bit of the marinade over the top, and grill for about 4 minutes, or until the chicken meat is completely white and the juices run clear. Serve with Peanut Sauce on the side.

Preparation time: *20 minutes*
Cooking time: *15 minutes for the Peanut Sauce; 5–6 minutes on a grill; 4 minutes in an electric grilling machine*
Makes 4 main-course servings (2 kabobs each); 16 appetizers

Nutritional Breakdown (per serving—based on main-course servings)

Calories: 796	*Carbohydrates: 43 gm*	*Cholesterol: 73 mg*	*Saturated fat: 18 gm*
Protein: 46 gm	*Sodium: 1211 mg*	*Fat: 54 gm*	*% calories fat: 58%*

Grilled Chicken Thighs over Acapulco Salad

Crispy salad, loaded with texture and flavor, and a juicy chicken thigh right off the grill make an ideal main course for a warm summer day. Grilled polenta or cornbread is a nice complement.

Chicken Marinade

¼ cup extra-virgin olive oil

¼ cup balsamic vinegar

2 tablespoons fresh lime juice

1 tablespoon honey

1 tablespoon chopped fresh rosemary, stemmed, or ½ tablespoon dried

2 garlic cloves, minced

Dash of chili powder

Grilled Chicken Thighs

4–6 skinless, boneless roasting-chicken thighs

Canola oil for the grid, if using a grill

Acapulco Salad

1 (8 ¾ ounce) can kidney beans, drained

1 avocado, peeled, seeded, and chopped

½ cup ripe, pitted, sliced black olives

¼ cup chopped green onions

3 cups green leaf or iceberg lettuce, torn in bite-size pieces

¼ cup salsa (page 66)

¼ cup reduced-fat mayonnaise*

¼ cup shredded reduced-fat white Cheddar cheese

1 cup crushed corn tortilla chips

1. To make the marinade, combine all the ingredients in a medium bowl, add the chicken thighs, and marinate for 2 to 6 hours.
2. Drain the chicken thighs and reserve the marinade for basting. Let the chicken sit at room temperature for 30 minutes before grilling.
3. Prepare the grill or electric grilling machine for cooking.

*You may substitute ½ cup storebought reduced-calorie taco dressing for the salsa and mayonnaise.

4. If using a charcoal grill, oil the grid and place it above ashen coals. Place the thighs, meaty side down, over direct heat and close the lid. Turn and baste frequently so the meat won't become dry. Cook until golden brown, about 8 to 10 minutes, or until no pink remains and the juices run clear.

5. If using an electric grilling machine, place the thighs on a hot grill and cook for 3 to 4 minutes, or until no pink remains and the juices run clear.

To prepare the salad:

1. Place the kidney beans, avocado, black olives, and green onions in a large salad bowl, and add the torn lettuce on top. Cover with a damp paper towel and refrigerate until ready to serve.

2. In a small bowl, combine the salsa and mayonnaise (unless you are using store-bought taco dressing).

3. Just before serving, toss the salad with the dressing. Serve on individual plates and top each plate with shredded cheese, crushed tortilla chips, and a grilled chicken thigh. Serve immediately.

Preparation time: *15–20 minutes*
Cooking time: *8–10 minutes on a grill; 3–4 minutes in an electric grilling machine*
Makes 4–6 servings

Nutritional Breakdown (per serving, based on 4 servings)

Calories: 716	*Carbohydrates: 65 gm*	*Cholesterol: 70 mg*	*Saturated fat: 8 gm*
Protein: 32 gm	*Sodium: 800 mg*	*Fat: 38 gm*	*% calories fat: 47%*

Rosemary-Thyme Chicken Strips over Lemon-Garlic Caesar Salad

This tangy main-course salad is a breeze to fix on a busy night. Served with crusty bread, it makes a complete and nourishing meal.

3 small boneless, skinless chicken breasts, cut into 1½-inch strips
1 recipe Rosemary-Thyme Marinade (see page 35)

6 bamboo skewers soaked in water 15–30 minutes, if using a grill
Canola oil for the grid, if using a grill

1. Place the chicken pieces in a shallow bowl and cover with marinade; turn the pieces several times to make sure all are coated with the marinade. Marinate in the refrigerator for 2 to 6 hours. Let stand for 30 minutes at room temperature before grilling.
2. While the chicken is marinating, prepare Lemon-Garlic Caesar Salad (page 131).
3. Prepare the grill or electric grilling machine for cooking.
4. If using a charcoal grill, thread the skewers with chicken pieces. Place the skewers on the grid over ashen coals and grill for about 9 minutes, or until the chicken is no longer pink and the juices run clear, turning and basting every 3 minutes.
5. If using an electric grilling machine, place the chicken pieces on a hot grill and cook for 1½ to 2 minutes, or until the meat is no longer pink and the juices run clear.
6. To serve, arrange the chicken pieces decoratively over each salad and top with Parmesan cheese and croutons or toasted sunflower seeds.

Preparation time: *10 minutes*
Cooking time: *about 9 minutes on a grill; 1½–2 minutes in an electric grilling machine*
Makes 4 servings

Nutritional Breakdown (per serving)

Calories: 336	*Carbohydrates: 1 gm*	*Cholesterol: 110 mg*	*Saturated fat: 3 gm*
Protein: 40 gm	*Sodium: 95 mg*	*Fat: 18 gm*	*% calories fat: 50%*

Lemon-Garlic Caesar Salad

You'll never miss raw egg yolk in this Caesar salad—it's so packed with zesty flavor. It's also abundant in nutrients. The lemon provides vitamin C, and the leafy greens, beta-carotene.

Salad

1 large head romaine lettuce, washed, dried, and torn into bite-size pieces

1 head Boston (Bibb) lettuce, washed, dried, and torn into bite-size pieces
1 clove garlic

Dressing

¾ cup fresh lemon juice, preferably juiced by hand
4 tablespoons red or white wine vinegar
1 (2 ounce) can anchovy fillets (optional)
3 cloves garlic, pressed

1 teaspoon Dijon mustard
3 dashes Worcestershire sauce
Salt and pepper to taste (optional)
1 cup extra-virgin olive oil

Toppings

½ cup freshly grated Parmesan cheese

Croutons or toasted sunflower seeds*

1. Tear the lettuce into a wooden salad bowl that has been rubbed with a crushed clove of garlic.
2. To make the dressing, put the lemon juice, vinegar, anchovies, if using, garlic, mustard, Worcestershire sauce, and salt and pepper, if using, in a blender or food processor with a steel blade, and process for 1 minute. (Though optional, anchovies do help to thicken the dressing and also add flavor.) Drizzle in the olive oil drop by drop until the dressing begins to thicken and then slowly drizzle in the remaining oil. (This makes about 3 cups of dressing and should last in the refrigerator for a couple of weeks.)

*To toast the seeds, place them on a baking sheet with a raised edge, and toast at 250° F for about 20 minutes, or until they are golden. Be careful not to burn them. They will become crunchier and more flavorful as they cool.

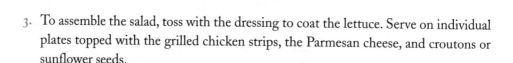

3. To assemble the salad, toss with the dressing to coat the lettuce. Serve on individual plates topped with the grilled chicken strips, the Parmesan cheese, and croutons or sunflower seeds.

Preparation time: *20 minutes*
Makes 4 servings

Nutritional Breakdown (per serving with 2 tablespoons dressing)

Calories: 157	*Carbohydrates: 4 gm*	*Cholesterol: 9 mg*	*Saturated fat: 4 gm*
Protein: 7 gm	*Sodium: 243 mg*	*Fat: 13 gm*	*% calories fat: 72%*

Nutribite

Main-course salads topped with a small serving of grilled poultry or meat represent a very healthful style of eating. In this way you can serve less animal protein and more high-fiber, nutrient-packed foods like vegetables with no one feeling deprived. The current recommendation from the United States Department of Agriculture is that we not consume more than 3 to 4 ounces of animal protein at a meal. Meat- or poultry-topped salads can help you and your family stay within these guidelines by pleasing your taste buds, providing some of the vegetable servings you're striving for (3 to 5 per day), and satisfying even the healthiest of appetites. Just ask me!

Knock-Out-the-Fat Tacos ♡

You can make tacos much lower in fat by using ground chicken or turkey instead of beef, adding chopped vegetables, and topping them with a reduced-fat sour cream sauce. With a few simple changes, you can knock the fat nearly in half, as evidenced by our recipe, which earned the heart-healthy symbol.

Tacos

1 pound ground, skinless chicken or turkey
    breast
¹/₂ cup minced onion
¹/₂ cup minced green or red bell pepper
1 teaspoon chili powder
¹/₂ teaspoon dried oregano
¹/₂ teaspoon ground cumin

¹/₄ teaspoon paprika
¹/₄ teaspoon freshly ground black pepper
1 garlic clove, minced
3–4 tablespoons taco sauce (optional)
12 crisp corn taco shells or soft corn or flour
    tortillas

Topping Options

Cilantro–Sour Cream Sauce
Shredded lettuce
Chopped tomatoes

Chopped onions
Shredded reduced-fat cheese
Salsa (page 66)

Cilantro–Sour Cream Sauce

4 tablespoons reduced-fat sour cream
4 tablespoons plain nonfat yogurt

2 tablespoons chopped fresh cilantro

1. To make the tacos, place the ground chicken or turkey, onion, bell pepper, chili powder, oregano, cumin, paprika, pepper, and garlic in a medium bowl, and mix well until all the ingredients are well combined.
2. To make the sour cream sauce, place all the ingredients in a small bowl, mix well, and chill.
3. Prepare the electric grilling machine for cooking. (Taco meat cannot be cooked on an outdoor grill.)
4. Put the ground chicken or turkey mixture on a hot grilling machine and cook for about 3 minutes, or until no pink remains and the juices run clear. Put the mixture in a medium-size bowl, add the taco sauce, if using, and mix well.

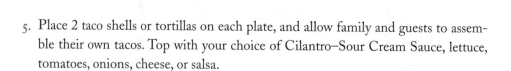

5. Place 2 taco shells or tortillas on each plate, and allow family and guests to assemble their own tacos. Top with your choice of Cilantro–Sour Cream Sauce, lettuce, tomatoes, onions, cheese, or salsa.

Preparation time: *10 minutes*
Cooking time: *about 3 minutes*
Makes 6 servings (2 tacos each)

Nutritional Breakdown (per serving)

Calories: 275	*Carbohydrates: 19 gm*	*Cholesterol: 46 mg*	*Saturated fat: 1 gm*
Protein: 19 gm	*Sodium: 141 mg*	*Fat: 8 gm*	*% calories fat: 30%*

Grilled Turkey Cutlets
with Honey-Dijon-Rosemary Marinade

Rich and flavorful, these turkey cutlets taste like you've been working in the kitchen for hours. The surprise is they can be made in minutes. Just allow at least 2 to 6 hours for marinating so the turkey can absorb all the great flavorings. Serve the cutlets over a bed of brown rice or linguine, heat the remaining marinade, and drizzle some over the top for a truly gourmet entrée. Or serve the cutlets over Caesar salad (page 131) for a great variation on a main-course salad.

Honey-Dijon-Rosemary Marinade

¼ cup extra-virgin olive oil
¼ cup white vinegar
¼ cup sherry
2 tablespoons honey
2 tablespoons Dijon mustard

2 tablespoons chopped fresh rosemary, stemmed
¼ teaspoon freshly ground black pepper
2 garlic cloves, minced

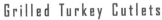

Grilled Turkey Cutlets

1 (3 to 4 pound) turkey breast, skinned, sliced with the grain into cutlets, and pounded (makes about 12 cutlets)

Canola oil for the grid, if using a grill

1. In a medium bowl, combine all the marinade ingredients, mixing well.
2. Place the turkey cutlets in a medium bowl and pour the marinade over the top, making sure the cutlets are well covered. Marinate, covered, in the refrigerator for 2 to 6 hours. Allow the turkey to sit at room temperature for about 30 minutes before grilling.
3. Prepare the grill or electric grilling machine for cooking.
4. If using a grill, place the cutlets on an oiled grid above ashen coals, cover, and cook for about 6 minutes, or until no pink remains, turning once and basting occasionally with marinade. Be careful not to overcook or the meat will be tough. Serve immediately.
5. If using an electric grilling machine, place the cutlets on a hot grill, drizzle a bit of the marinade over the top, and cook for about 3 minutes, or until the meat is no longer pink. Serve immediately.

Preparation time: *10 minutes*
Cooking time: *about 6 minutes on a grill; about 3 minutes in an electric grilling machine*
Makes 6 servings

Nutritional Breakdown (per serving)

Calories: 330	*Carbohydrates: 4 gm*	*Cholesterol: 138 mg*	*Saturated fat: 2 gm*
Protein: 51 gm	*Sodium: 182 mg*	*Fat: 10 gm*	*% calories fat: 30%*

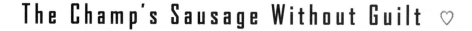

The Champ's Sausage Without Guilt ♡

〰 Start your day with a sausage patty that's good for you. This moist, flavorful turkey sausage, served with a country-style biscuit, makes a complete breakfast meal. (This recipe is from Cherie's book *The Healthy Gourmet,* published by Clarkson Potter.)

1 slightly beaten egg white
⅓ cup minced onion
¼ cup finely chopped dried apples or
   ½ cup chopped fresh sweet apples
¼ cup seasoned bread crumbs
2 tablespoons snipped fresh parsley
½ teaspoon salt (optional)

½ teaspoon crushed sage
¼ teaspoon ground nutmeg
¼ teaspoon ground black pepper
Pinch cayenne pepper
½ pound lean, ground, skinless turkey
   breast
Canola oil for the grid, if using a grill

1. In a medium bowl, combine the egg white, onion, dried or fresh apples, bread crumbs, parsley, salt, if using, sage, nutmeg, black pepper, and cayenne pepper. Add the ground turkey and mix well.
2. With moistened fingers, shape the mixture into eight 2-inch patties.
3. Prepare the grill or electric grilling machine for cooking.
4. If using a charcoal grill, place the patties on an oiled grid over ashen coals and grill for 8 to 10 minutes, or until the meat is no longer pink, turning once.
5. If using an electric grilling machine, place the patties on a hot grill and cook for 3 to 4 minutes, or until the meat is no longer pink.

Preparation time: *5 minutes*
Cooking time: *8–10 minutes on a grill; 3–4 minutes in an electric grilling machine*
Makes 4 servings (2 patties each)

Nutritional Breakdown (per serving)

Calories: 115	Carbohydrates: 9 gm	Cholesterol: 34 mg	Saturated fat: 0 gm
Protein: 15 gm	Sodium: 247 mg	Fat: 2 gm	% calories fat: 14%

Nutribite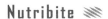

Choose ground skinless turkey breast over ground dark turkey meat and skin for lowest fat. For a 3-ounce serving, you'll save over 50 calories and reduce the fat from 11 to 3 grams. Turkey, and especially the light meat, is a good source of niacin, an important B vitamin needed to maintain a healthy nervous system. It is also an excellent source of tryptophan, an amino acid that helps promote restful sleep.

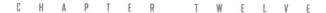

PORK

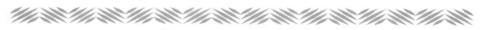

THERE'S NOTHING LIKE OLD-FASHIONED BARBECUED PORK RIBS for mouth-watering enjoyment. Sweet and tender, pork absorbs the flavors of marinades readily and stays moist during cooking. Most cuts can be grilled directly over heat. Ribs are a traditional favorite for barbecuing, which should be done slowly over indirect heat. Pork accepts the sweet, tangy flavors of barbecue sauce well. It is also ideal for barbecuing because there is enough internal fat to keep it moist and juicy during cooking.

Pork chops and tenderloin are excellent for grilling, but most cuts grill well. Spareribs, country-style ribs, baby back ribs, pork shoulder, and pork butt are all excellent barbecued. Ribs, a rather tough meat, should always be cooked slowly over a drip pan. This enables them to become tender and succulent. Country-style ribs are the rib end of the pork loin and are very good when marinated first. They are excellent served with John's Hot and Spicy Rub for Ribs (page 40) and South Carolina Mustard Sauce (page 44).

Whenever possible, choose pork with a label that says it was raised *naturally,* meaning without the use of antibiotics, hormones, steroids, growth stimulants, or any other drugs. Also, pigs that are allowed to roam freely, rather than being confined to small pens, will be the healthiest animals. And the healthiest animals produce the healthiest meat.

When it comes to how often you eat pork, we recommend that you choose it only for special occasions. Despite its recent PR as "the other white meat," pork is high in saturated fat and has to be cooked very well to kill any parasites that may be in it.

TIPS FOR GRILLING AND BARBECUING PORK

1. Always cook pork well done, to about 145° F, but be careful not to overcook it or it will be dried out and tough.

2. If it can be avoided, don't freeze pork. Pork's cell walls tend to break down easily during freezing, causing water loss and, thus, a drier piece of meat.

3. Always cook ribs over low, indirect heat using a drip pan until they can be pulled apart easily. Avoid boiling ribs beforehand.

4. Wait until the ribs are at least half cooked before basting them with a tomato-based sauce, since the sauce may burn before the ribs are done.

5. Cook a slab of ribs whole and cut them when done. This will keep the meat juicy.

6. If raw pork meat was marinated, always cook the marinade sauce very well before serving.

7. Always wash the platter on which you carried raw meat to the grill in hot, soapy water before using it to serve the cooked pork or other food.

The Foreman Family Breakfast Sausage

Early in the morning when the kids request pork sausage patties, I cook them. I love to make sausage on the grill because it's great to see so much fat disappear. And you can really see it run off my grilling machine! Sausage patties cook best in an electric grilling machine, but they can also be done on an outdoor grill. This sausage is delicious served with French toast.

1 pound ground pork
3 tablespoons water
2 teaspoons fennel seeds
2 teaspoons crushed sage
2 teaspoons freshly ground black pepper

1½ teaspoons ground ginger
1 teaspoon poultry seasoning
½ teaspoon salt (optional)
Canola oil for the grid, if using a grill

1. In a medium bowl, combine all the ingredients and mix with your fingers until the ingredients are well combined. Form the mixture into ten 2-inch patties.
2. Prepare the grill or electric grilling machine for cooking.
3. If using a charcoal grill, oil the grid and place it above ashen coals. Grill the sausage patties directly above the heat for 2 to 3 minutes on each side, or until the juices run clear and no pink remains.
4. If using an electric grilling machine, place the sausage patties on a hot grill and cook for about 4 minutes, or until the juices run clear and no pink remains.

Preparation time: *5 minutes*
Cooking time: *4–6 minutes on a grill; about 4 minutes in an electric grilling machine*
Makes about 5 servings (2 patties each)

Nutritional Breakdown (per serving)

Calories: 183	Carbohydrates: 2 gm	Cholesterol: 56 mg	Saturated fat: 5 gm
Protein: 16 gm	Sodium: 51 mg	Fat: 12 gm	% calories fat: 60%

Stuffed Pork Chops
with Honey-Pineapple Marinade

Thick, juicy stuffed pork chops are ideal fare for an early-fall grill when the nights are cooler. These hearty pork chops need only a green salad and seasoned vegetables to complete a casual supper for four. They are the most flavorful when marinated for 4 hours to overnight.

Honey-Pineapple Marinade

¼ cup light soy sauce or tamari

¼ cup white vinegar

¼ cup extra-virgin olive oil

¼ cup fresh or canned (packed in juice) crushed pineapple

2 tablespoons honey

2 tablespoons minced ginger

2 garlic cloves, minced

Pork Chops

4 pork chops, center cut, ¾ pound each, for the grill; boneless center cut or boneless pork loin (about ½–1 inch thick) for an electric grilling machine

Wooden toothpicks for closing pork chop pockets

Canola oil for the grid, if using a grill

Stuffing

2 teaspoons butter

2 teaspoons extra-virgin olive oil

1 cup chopped onion

1 cup chopped celery

1 teaspoon crushed sage

½ teaspoon dried rosemary

½ teaspoon dried basil

½ teaspoon dried oregano

½ teaspoon freshly ground black pepper

8 slices whole-wheat bread, toasted, cut into cubes

¼ cup fresh or canned (packed in juice) crushed pineapple

1 cup chicken broth

2 eggs

Salt to taste (optional)

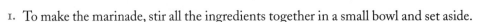
1. To make the marinade, stir all the ingredients together in a small bowl and set aside.
2. Cut a pocket in each pork chop and trim away the extra fat. Place the pork chops in a shallow dish and cover with the marinade, allowing the marinade to seep inside the pockets. Marinate in the refrigerator for 4 hours to overnight.
3. To make the stuffing, in a large skillet, melt the butter over medium-high heat and add the olive oil. Sauté the onion, celery, sage, rosemary, basil, oregano, and pepper until the onion is translucent, about 10 minutes. Reduce the heat to low, add the bread and crushed pineapple, and cook for 1 minute. Add the chicken broth and cook for another minute.
4. Transfer the stuffing to a large mixing bowl, add the eggs (and salt, if using) and mix well.
5. Drain the pork chops, reserving the marinade, and stuff each with bread stuffing. Close each pocket with toothpicks to hold the stuffing inside.
6. Prepare the grill or electric grilling machine for cooking.
7. If using a charcoal grill, oil the grid and place it above ashen coals. Place the chops directly above the heat and grill for 10 to 12 minutes, basting occasionally with the remaining marinade. Turn and cook, basting occasionally, for another 10 to 12 minutes, or until nicely browned and cooked thoroughly. Juices should run clear when a chop is pierced with a fork at the thickest part, and no pink should remain. Serve immediately.
8. If using an electric grilling machine, place the chops on a hot grill and cook for 5 to 7 minutes, or until nicely browned and cooked thoroughly. Juices should run clear when a chop is pierced with a fork at the thickest part, and no pink should remain. Serve immediately.

Preparation time: *30 minutes*
Cooking time: *27–31 minutes on a grill; 5–7 minutes for boneless chops in an electric grilling machine*
Makes 4 servings

Nutritional Breakdown (per serving)

Calories: 505	*Carbohydrates: 38 gm*	*Cholesterol: 180 mg*	*Saturated fat: 7 gm*
Protein: 31 gm	*Sodium: 873 mg*	*Fat: 26 gm*	*% calories fat: 46%*

Nutribite 〰

Keep in mind that a thick center-cut pork chop will be far more meat than the USDA Food Guide Pyramid recommendation of 3 to 4 ounces per serving. So when you want to splurge with our stuffed pork chops, we suggest cutting back at another time during the week with a light supper, such as a vegetarian dish like the Vegetarian Kabobs (page 163) or the Barbecued Tofu (page 162).

Grilled Pork Chops
with Sage-Wine Marinade

〰 Sage is an ideal complement to pork and is used often with roast pork. It lends distinct flavor to this pork grill. An ideal accompaniment is warm cinnamon applesauce.

Sage-Wine Marinade

¼ cup extra-virgin olive oil
¼ cup herbed vinegar
¼ cup white wine
1 tablespoon honey

2 teaspoons crushed sage
¼ teaspoon freshly ground black pepper
2 garlic cloves, minced

Grilled Pork Chops

4 pork loin chops, about ½ inch thick (center-cut boneless pork loin chops work best in an electric grilling machine)

Canola oil for the grid, if using a grill

1. To make the marinade, combine all the ingredients in a medium bowl and mix well.
2. Place the pork chops in a shallow dish and pour the marinade over the top. Cover and marinate in the refrigerator for 4 hours to overnight, turning once or twice. Let the chops stand at room temperature for 30 minutes before grilling. Reserve the marinade.
3. Prepare the grill or electric grilling machine for cooking.

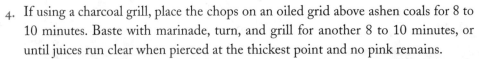

4. If using a charcoal grill, place the chops on an oiled grid above ashen coals for 8 to 10 minutes. Baste with marinade, turn, and grill for another 8 to 10 minutes, or until juices run clear when pierced at the thickest point and no pink remains.

5. If using an electric grilling machine, place the chops on a hot grill and cook for 5 to 7 minutes, depending on the thickness and if they are boneless. When done, they should be lightly firm to the touch, the juices should run clear when pierced at the thickest point, and no pink should remain.

Preparation time: *5 minutes*
Cooking time: *16–20 minutes on a grill; 5–7 minutes for boneless chops in an electric grilling machine*
Makes 4 servings

Nutritional Breakdown (per serving)

Calories: 255	*Carbohydrates: 3 gm*	*Cholesterol: 68 mg*	*Saturated fat: 4 gm*
Protein: 21 gm	*Sodium: 52 mg*	*Fat: 17 gm*	*% calories fat: 59%*

Country-Style Ribs
with Louisiana Bacon Barbecue Sauce

Meaty country-style pork ribs and crunchy bacon barbecue sauce make this barbecue an "event." Add the Barbecued Sweet Potato–Apple Kabobs (page 156) basted with the sauce and make a meal to remember.

Louisiana Bacon Barbecue Sauce

¾ cup chopped bacon
½ cup chopped onion
½ cup chopped green bell pepper
2 garlic cloves, minced
1 (10 ¾ ounce) can tomato puree
½ cup honey
¼ cup chicken broth
2 tablespoons chili powder

1 tablespoon freshly grated orange zest
1 tablespoon freshly grated lemon zest
1 teaspoon cayenne pepper
¼ teaspoon freshly ground black pepper
1 teaspoon butter
Juice of ½ orange
Juice of ½ lemon

Country-Style Pork Ribs

8 country-style pork ribs (about 4 pounds)*
Canola oil for the grid, if using a grill

To make the barbecue sauce:

1. In a medium saucepan over medium-high heat, cook the bacon until crisp, 5 to 6 minutes.
2. Remove the bacon and drain on paper towels. Pour off all but 2 tablespoons of the bacon grease.
3. Reduce the heat to medium and sauté the onion, bell pepper, and garlic until tender, about 10 minutes.
4. Add the tomato puree, honey, chicken broth, chili powder, orange and lemon zests, cayenne pepper, black pepper, butter, and orange and lemon juices, and stir well.

* Thick, meaty ribs do not cook well in an electric grilling machine. For thick country-style ribs, we recommend outdoor grilling; however, thin-sliced country-style pork ribs will work in an electric griller. Ask your butcher to slice country-style ribs thin if not available at your market.

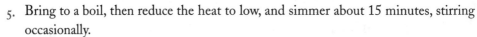

5. Bring to a boil, then reduce the heat to low, and simmer about 15 minutes, stirring occasionally.

6. Stir in the bacon, and if you want a smooth sauce, pour the mixture into a blender or food processor with a steel blade and process until the bacon is finely chopped. Return the mixture to a saucepan and keep warm until ready to serve. Serve as a finishing and table sauce.

7. The sauce can be refrigerated for up to a week or frozen. (If frozen, add 2 to 4 tablespoons of water to reconstitute.)

To barbecue the ribs:

1. Prepare the grill for cooking.

2. If using a charcoal grill, oil the grid and place it above ashen coals. Brown the ribs directly over the coals on both sides, allowing about 5 minutes per side. Then move the ribs over a drip pan, bone side down. Baste the ribs with sauce and close the lid. Baste about every 10 minutes. After 30 minutes flip the ribs over, basting and flipping every 10 minutes until done. Ribs should be done in about 1 hour.

3. If using an electric grilling machine, cook as many of the thin-sliced country-style ribs as will fit on a hot grill at one time. Baste with sauce and cook until done, about 4 to 5 minutes.

4. Serve with hot barbecue sauce on the side.

Preparation time: *10 minutes*

Cooking time: *about 20 minutes for the sauce; about 1 hour on a grill; 4–5 minutes for thin-sliced, country-style ribs in an electric grilling machine*

Makes 4 servings (2 ribs each)

Nutritional Breakdown (per serving)

Calories: 1131	*Carbohydrates: 51 gm*	*Cholesterol: 214 mg*	*Saturated fat: 19 gm*
Protein: 104 gm	*Sodium: 765 mg*	*Fat: 56 gm*	*% calories fat: 45%*

Nutribite

This recipe delivers a double helping of pork with the thick country-style ribs and the bacon in the sauce. For health's sake, we recommend this meal for only a special occasion.

Southeast Asian Spareribs

The marinade imbues ribs with fabulous flavor as well as tenderizing them. Serve these spareribs with rice noodles and a sweet grated carrot salad for an authentic Southeast Asian meal.

Marinade

⅔ cup honey
⅓ cup light soy sauce or tamari
¼ cup toasted sesame oil
2 tablespoons sesame seeds

1 tablespoon rice vinegar
1 teaspoon dry mustard
¼ teaspoon freshly ground black pepper

Spareribs

3½–4 pounds spareribs (have the butcher crack the "wing" of the spareribs, so that after cooking you can cut them easily between the bones)

*Canola oil for the grid, if using the grill**

1. To make the marinade, combine all the ingredients in a shallow bowl. Add the ribs and turn them in the marinade to cover on all sides. Cover and refrigerate for 8 to 12 hours.
2. Remove the ribs from the marinade and blot off the excess marinade. Reserve the marinade.
3. Prepare the grill or the electric grilling machine for cooking.
4. If using a charcoal grill, oil the grid and place it above ashen coals. Brown the ribs over direct heat, about 3 minutes on each side. Then place the ribs over indirect heat using a drip pan and close the lid. Baste the ribs with marinade and turn about every 15 minutes until done. Ribs are done when the meat begins to fall off the bone, about 45 minutes. Allow the ribs to sit about 5 minutes to retain their juices before slicing.

* *Spareribs are not appropriate for an electric grilling machine; thin-sliced, country-style pork ribs can be substituted in this recipe. Ask your butcher to slice ribs thin if not available at your market.*

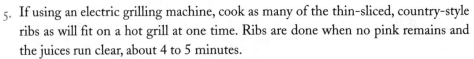

5. If using an electric grilling machine, cook as many of the thin-sliced, country-style ribs as will fit on a hot grill at one time. Ribs are done when no pink remains and the juices run clear, about 4 to 5 minutes.

6. Serve with hot marinade on the side. (Be sure to heat the marinade thoroughly before serving because of the raw meat that marinated in it.)

Preparation time: *5 minutes*

Cooking time: *45 minutes on a grill; 4–5 minutes for thin-sliced, country-style ribs in an electric grilling machine*

Makes 3–4 servings

Nutritional Breakdown (per serving)

Calories: 889	*Carbohydrates: 19 gm*	*Cholesterol: 209 mg*	*Saturated fat: 19 gm*
Protein: 84 gm	*Sodium: 533 mg*	*Fat: 51 gm*	*% calories fat: 53%*

Pork and Pineapple Skewers
with Ginger-Sesame Marinade

The pork is bathed in an Asian-style sauce that blends a delightful combination of ginger and sesame. Serve the kabobs with short-grain brown or jasmine rice with the marinade on the side. Be sure to heat the marinade thoroughly before serving because of the raw meat that marinated in it.

Ginger-Sesame Marinade

¼ cup extra-virgin olive oil
¼ cup light soy sauce or tamari
2 tablespoons toasted sesame oil
2 tablespoons sesame seeds

1 tablespoon minced ginger
1 teaspoon chili powder
2 garlic cloves, minced

Pork and Pineapple Skewers

3–4 boneless pork cutlets, cut into 1-inch
*   chunks (about 1 pound)*
¼ fresh pineapple, peeled and cut into
*   1-inch chunks (canned pineapple can*
*   be substituted)*

16 green onions, trimmed and cut, with
*   2 inches of green remaining*
8 bamboo skewers, soaked in water for
*   15–30 minutes*
Canola oil for the grid, if using a grill

1. To prepare the marinade, mix all the ingredients in a small bowl, add the pork chunks, cover, and marinate in the refrigerator for 4 hours to overnight.
2. About 1 hour before serving, drain the pork, reserving the marinade. If using an electric grilling machine, cut the bamboo skewers to fit the length of the machine. Thread the pork, pineapple chunks, and green onions alternately on skewers and place them in a shallow bowl. Baste the kabobs with some of the marinade and let them sit at room temperature for about 30 minutes before grilling.
3. Prepare the grill or electric grilling machine for cooking.
4. If using a charcoal grill, oil the grid and place it above ashen coals. Place the skewers directly over the heat, turning and basting frequently for about 12 minutes, or until the pork is thoroughly cooked—no pink remains and the juices run clear.

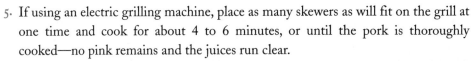

5. If using an electric grilling machine, place as many skewers as will fit on the grill at one time and cook for about 4 to 6 minutes, or until the pork is thoroughly cooked—no pink remains and the juices run clear.

6. To serve, place 2 skewers on each plate over a bed of rice and serve the marinade hot as a sauce on the side. (Be sure to heat the marinade thoroughly because raw meat has been marinating in it.)

Preparation time: *10–15 minutes*
Cooking time: *about 12 minutes on the grill; 4–6 minutes in an electric grilling machine*
Makes 4 servings (2 skewers each)

Nutritional Breakdown (per person)

Calories: 264	*Carbohydrates: 7 gm*	*Cholesterol: 51 mg*	*Saturated fat: 4 gm*
Protein: 17 gm	*Sodium: 355 mg*	*Fat: 19 gm*	*% calories fat: 63%*

Nutribite

Pineapple is an excellent source of the protein-digesting enzyme bromelain, which helps promote better digestion. Many studies have shown that bromelain assists the body's response to inflammation and swelling, which makes it excellent for arthritis sufferers.

Ginger Pork Salad

A great main course or side salad, this dish can be prepared a day ahead and refrigerated until ready to serve. Actually, it becomes more flavorful if it sits for a while, as this allows the rice and pork to absorb the dressing.

2 boneless pork-loin chops
Canola oil for the chops and the grid, if
    using a grill
3 cups cooked brown rice
1/4 pound fresh or frozen (thawed) snow
    peas, trimmed and cut into slivers
1 medium cucumber, peeled, seeded, and cut
    into slivers
1 red bell pepper, cut into slivers

1/2 cup chopped green onions
2 tablespoons minced ginger
2 tablespoons toasted sesame seeds*
1/4 cup chicken broth
3 tablespoons rice vinegar
3 tablespoons light soy sauce or tamari
1 tablespoon peanut oil
2 teaspoons toasted sesame oil

1. Prepare the grill or electric grilling machine for cooking.
2. If using a charcoal grill, oil the grid and place it above ashen coals. Brush the chops with oil and place them directly over the heat. Grill for about 8 to 10 minutes, turning frequently, or until the meat is lightly firm to the touch, the juices run clear, and no pink remains. Remove and slice into thin, bite-size strips.
3. If using an electric grilling machine, place the pork chops on a hot grill and cook for 5 to 7 minutes.
4. In a large bowl, combine the rice, pork, snow peas, cucumber, bell pepper, green onions, ginger, and sesame seeds.
5. In a small jar with a lid, combine the chicken broth, vinegar, soy sauce or tamari, peanut oil, and sesame oil. Shake and pour over the rice mixture, and toss lightly. Serve chilled.

* Place the sesame seeds in a small cast-iron skillet and bake at 250° F for about 20 minutes, or until they are golden, being careful not to burn them. Remove from the oven and cool; they will get crunchier and more flavorful as they cool.

Preparation time: *15 minutes*
Cooking time: *8–10 minutes on a grill; 4–7 minutes in an electric grilling machine*
Makes 6 servings

Nutritional Breakdown (per serving)

Calories: 242	*Carbohydrates: 28 gm*	*Cholesterol: 23 mg*	*Saturated fat: 2 gm*
Protein: 12 gm	*Sodium: 365 mg*	*Fat: 10 gm*	*% calories fat: 35%*

Nutribite ≋

Gingerroot not only adds flavor, but also has therapeutic benefits. Scientific studies show that this pungent, aromatic herb has anti-inflammatory properties, can help prevent motion sickness, thins the blood, lowers cholesterol, and helps in preventing cancer.

VEGETABLES AND VEGETARIAN BARBECUE

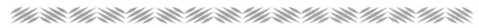

FLAVORFUL AND COLORFUL, GRILLED VEGETABLES LEND THEIR beauty to any meal. Your choices are limited only by your imagination. Any vegetable can be cooked on the grill. Just watch them so they don't burn. Or they can be wrapped in aluminum-foil "tents," with some marinade or salad dressing drizzled over the top for a delicious variation. Vegetables can also be barbecued—cooked slowly over a drip pan while you're doing the entrée (although they'll take less time than meat or chicken) and brushed near the end with a little barbecue sauce.

Timing is important for vegetables, especially when it comes to kabobs or a variety of vegetables on the grill. In order for all the vegetables to be done at the same time, those that take the longest to cook will have to be started first. Or you can parboil the ones that take the longest (bell peppers and onions, for example) before grilling or threading them onto skewers.

Grilling is a delicious way to introduce vegetarian dishes into your diet and perhaps convert a few nonvegetarians. Everyone loves the flavors that come from grilling. Tofu never tastes so good as when it's grilled or barbecued with your favorite sauce. Different types of veggie burgers are fabulous when served with all the trimmings, and unless you tell your family what they are, they may not even notice you didn't serve red meat in the buns.

Whenever possible, choose vegetables that are *organically grown*, meaning without the use of synthetic pesticides, herbicides, and fertilizers. Your body will thank you over the years with better health.

TIPS FOR GRILLING AND BARBECUING VEGETABLES AND TOFU

1. Be careful not to overcook vegetables when grilling; watch them closely.

2. The simplest way to grill vegetables is to brush them with oil, then rub them with minced garlic and fresh herbs. Cook vegetables over direct heat alongside meat, poultry, or fish on an oiled grill.

3. Slice zucchini and eggplant lengthwise ½ inch thick.

4. If you want to add vegetables with meat, poultry, or fish onto skewers, select vegetables that will cook in about the same amount of time. For example, shrimp cooks very quickly, so the best choices would be cherry tomatoes, green onions, or mushrooms, which also cook quickly. Any meat that takes longer to cook goes well with vegetables like bell peppers, onions, or zucchini.

5. Before grilling or barbecuing tofu, always press the water out of the tofu using paper towels.

Vegetable Kabobs
with Raspberry Vinegar Marinade ♡

Vegetable kabobs are a nice accompaniment with any grilled meat, poultry, or fish entrée. Since the USDA recommends that we eat 3 to 5 servings of vegetables each day, kabobs make an attractive presentation for at least 1 of those servings.

2 onions, cut into 8 wedges
¼ green bell pepper, cut into squares
12 mushrooms, stemmed and washed
8 cherry tomatoes
1 zucchini, cut in ½-inch slices

Canola oil for the grid, if using a grill
4 bamboo skewers, soaked for 15–30
  minutes in water
1 recipe Raspberry Vinegar Marinade
  (page 35)

1. For more even cooking, first blanch the onions and green peppers for 5 to 6 minutes, since they take longer to cook.
2. Thread the skewers, alternating mushrooms, cherry tomatoes, onions, green peppers, and zucchini. (If using an electric grilling machine, cut the skewers to fit the grill.) Arrange the skewers in a dish and pour the marinade over them. Refrigerate for 3 hours to overnight.
3. Prepare the grill or grilling machine for cooking.
4. If using a charcoal grill, place the kabobs on an oiled grid over ashen coals. Brush with marinade, cover, and grill for 10 to 12 minutes, turning once and basting occasionally.
5. If using an electric grilling machine, brush the grill lightly with oil and place the kabobs on a hot grill. Drizzle a bit of the marinade over the kabobs, cover, and cook about 3 minutes, or until all the vegetables are tender.

Preparation time: *10 minutes*
Cooking time: *10–12 minutes on a grill; about 3 minutes in an electric grilling machine*
Makes 4 servings

Nutritional Breakdown (per serving)

Calories: 210	*Carbohydrates: 34 gm*	*Cholesterol: 0 mg*	*Saturated fat: 1 gm*
Protein: 4 gm	*Sodium: 124 mg*	*Fat: 7 gm*	*% calories fat: 29%*

Barbecued Sweet Potato– Apple Kabobs ♡

These sweet, spicy kabobs are very good served alongside any barbecued entrée, and they are especially delicious with Cherie's Barbecued Chicken with Apple-Cinnamon Sauce (page 116) or Country-Style Ribs with Louisiana Bacon Barbecue Sauce (page 145).

2 sweet potatoes or yams
2 apples, cored and cut into chunks
¼ cup barbecue sauce, prepared or home-made

8 bamboo skewers, soaked in water 15–30 minutes
Canola oil for the grid, if using a grill

1. Boil the sweet potatoes or yams for about 20 minutes, or until tender enough that a fork will pierce almost to the center. Peel and cut into chunks.
2. Alternately thread the sweet potato or yams and apple chunks onto skewers, starting and ending with potatoes.
3. Prepare the grill or electric grilling machine for cooking.
4. If using a charcoal grill, brush the grid with oil and place it above ashen coals. Place the kabobs on a part of the grill that is not over direct heat. Brush the top side with barbecue sauce and grill for about 10 minutes. Turn, brush with sauce, and cook for about another 5 minutes, or until the potatoes are tender in the center.
5. If using an electric grilling machine, brush both sides of the kabobs with barbecue sauce. Place the skewers on a hot grill and cook for 3 to 4 minutes, or until the potatoes are tender in the center.

Preparation time: *10 minutes*
Cooking time: *about 20 minutes to precook the potatoes; about 15 minutes on a grill; 3–4 minutes in an electric grilling machine*
Makes 4 servings (2 kabobs each)

Nutritional Breakdown (per serving)

Calories: 278	*Carbohydrates: 67 gm*	*Cholesterol: 0 mg*	*Saturated fat: 1 gm*
Protein: 3 gm	*Sodium: 296 mg*	*Fat: 3 gm*	*% calories fat: 8%*

Nutribite ≫

In scientific studies, yams and sweet potatoes have been shown to be particularly effective in helping to prevent cancer. They are rich in beta-carotene, a well-known anticancer factor. In addition, they are abundant sources of protease inhibitors, compounds that have been shown effective in halting cancer formation in animals. Protease inhibitors also help fight viruses.

Mixed Vegetable Grill with Balsamic Marinade

≫ A perfect accompaniment with fish, poultry, or meat, these vegetables are very easy to prepare and they taste *sooo* good. The marinade is made with balsamic vinegar, an Italian wine-based, aged vinegar. This marinade also makes a great salad dressing, and you should have enough left over to dress your greens.

Balsamic Marinade

¼ cup extra-virgin olive oil
¼ cup balsamic vinegar
1 tablespoon honey
2 teaspoons dried basil

1 teaspoon dried oregano
¼ teaspoon freshly ground black pepper
Juice of ½ lemon
Salt to taste

Vegetables

1 zucchini, cut lengthwise into 1-inch slices
1 onion, cut into chunks

1 red or green bell pepper, cut lengthwise into quarters; remove seeds, stem, and ribs
6–8 mushrooms, washed, dried, and halved

1. In a medium bowl, combine all the marinade ingredients and stir well. Set aside.
2. Make a "tent" with heavy aluminum foil as follows: Cut a large piece of foil and place the vegetables in the middle. Spoon several tablespoons of marinade over them. Pull the two sides together and roll down toward the center; roll the sides in toward the middle.

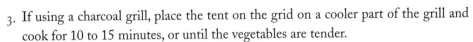

3. If using a charcoal grill, place the tent on the grid on a cooler part of the grill and cook for 10 to 15 minutes, or until the vegetables are tender.

4. If using an electric grilling machine, place the tent on a hot grill and cook for about 5 minutes, or until the vegetables are tender.

Preparation time: *10 minutes*
Cooking time: *10–15 minutes on a grill; 5 minutes in an electric grilling machine*
Makes 4 servings

Nutritional Breakdown (per serving)

Calories: 156	Carbohydrates: 22 gm	Cholesterol: 0 mg	Saturated fat: 1 gm
Protein: 3 gm	Sodium: 17 mg	Fat: 7 gm	% calories fat: 39%

Roasted New Potatoes with Garlic and Rosemary ♡

Roasted new potatoes go well with just about any grilled or barbecued food. Start the potatoes first, though, because they usually take the most time to cook. This recipe is so easy to make—wrap everything in foil, toss it on the grill. There's nothing to wash when you're done, and that's always good news.

8 new red potatoes or small purple potatoes,
*   scrubbed and cut in quarters*
2 green onions, chopped
2 garlic cloves, minced

1 sprig fresh rosemary, stems removed,
*   chopped*
1–2 tablespoons extra-virgin olive oil
Salt and pepper to taste

1. To make aluminum-foil "tents," lay a large piece of foil on the counter and place the potatoes in the center. Sprinkle green onions, garlic, and rosemary over them and drizzle olive oil on top. Add salt and pepper as desired.

2. Pull the middle pieces of the aluminum foil together and roll down toward the center. Then roll the ends toward the middle.

3. Prepare the grill or electric grilling machine for cooking.

4. If using a charcoal grill, place the aluminum-foil tent on the cooler portion of the grid over indirect heat, cover, and cook about 40 minutes, or until the potatoes are tender.

5. If using an electric grilling machine, place the aluminum-foil tent on a hot grill and cook for 12 to 15 minutes, or until the potatoes are tender.

Preparation time: *5 minutes*
Cooking time: *40 minutes on a grill; 12–15 minutes in an electric grilling machine*
Makes 4 servings

Nutritional Breakdown (per serving)

Calories: 143	*Carbohydrates: 26 gm*	*Cholesterol: 0 mg*	*Saturated fat: 0*
Protein: 3 gm	*Sodium: 8 mg*	*Fat: 3.5 gm*	*% calories fat: 22%*

Roasted Garlic

One of Cherie's favorite hors d'oeuvres is roasted garlic cloves, squeezed from their papery skins and spread over slices of French bread. Roasted garlic is a great complement to any grilled or barbecued meal.

6 heads garlic, unpeeled   *1 tablespoon butter*
¼ cup extra-virgin olive oil   *1 loaf French bread*

1. Prepare the grill. (This recipe will not work in an electric grilling machine.)

2. Cut the top part off the garlic heads, exposing the individual cloves. Place the heads on a piece of aluminum foil and drizzle with olive oil. Dot with butter and tightly seal the foil. Place the foil on a spot on the grill that is not directly over the coals.

3. After 40 minutes, open the foil and baste with the oil mixture. Reseal and roast until soft and spreadable, about 40 minutes.

4. Serve the garlic hot with French bread.

Preparation time: *2 minutes*
Cooking time: *about 1 hour and 20 minutes*
Makes 4–6 servings

Nutritional Breakdown (per serving)

Calories: 261	*Carbohydrates: 32 gm*	*Cholesterol: 5 mg*	*Saturated fat: 3 gm*
Protein: 6 gm	*Sodium: 326 mg*	*Fat: 13 gm*	*% calories fat: 43%*

Nutribite ≫

Over the centuries the reputation of the healing powers of garlic has been passed down by priests, physicians, and town healers. Today, there is research evidence that garlic has antibioticlike properties; fights infections; helps prevent cancer; reduces blood pressure, cholesterol, and triglycerides; and stimulates the immune system. When Cherie worked as a nutritionist at a medical center, one of her patients swore that two cloves of garlic, minced and swallowed with a glass of water, knocked out flu bugs overnight if taken early on. So Cherie tried it when she felt flu symptoms coming on, and by morning she felt much better. Ever since, at the Calbom house there's always been garlic hanging around.

Roasted Red Peppers

≫ The sweet, pungent flavor of roasted peppers enhances salads, stuffings, and grilled meats and poultry.

2 red bell peppers (orange or yellow can be substituted)

Olive oil for brushing the peppers and the grid of the grill

1. Wash the bell peppers and pat dry; brush with olive oil.
2. Prepare the grill. (Peppers cannot be roasted whole in an electric grilling machine.)
3. Place the peppers on an oiled grid directly over ashen coals. Turn the peppers often to char the skins; be careful not to burn them.

4. When the peppers are charred all over, remove them from the heat. Depending on the type of peppers and the thickness of the skins, the time can vary from 10 to 40 minutes.

5. Place the peppers in a sealable plastic bag or heavy paper bag for about 10 minutes to allow them to steam.

6. Place the peppers on a cutting board and allow them to cool enough to handle. Peel off the charred skin, scraping any stubborn areas with a knife. Then cut out the stems, slice the peppers down one side, remove the seeds and ribs, and place them in a bowl to collect the juices.

7. Serve immediately or store in a cool place, in a bowl covered with a little bit of additional olive oil.

Preparation time: *5 minutes*
Cooking time: *10–40 minutes*
Makes about ½ cup

Nutritional Breakdown (per serving)

Calories: 60	*Carbohydrates: 10 gm*	*Cholesterol: 0 mg*	*Saturated fat: 0 gm*
Protein: 1 gm	*Sodium: 3 mg*	*Fat: 2.5 gm*	*% calories fat: 34%*

Nutribite

Sweet red peppers are one of the richest sources of vitamin C; gram for gram they contain more than four times that found in oranges and orange juice. To help prevent colds and flu, get more vitamin C in your diet by including more bell peppers (red, green, yellow, orange, or purple), kale, parsley, broccoli, brussels sprouts, cauliflower, red cabbage, and strawberries. They're all loaded with this important antioxidant.

Barbecued Tofu

Cherie's friend Vicki Rae Chelf has devoted an entire cookbook to vegetarian barbecue. She sent me this recipe for a change of pace from Garden Burgers (page 61). (This recipe is adapted from *The Sensuous Vegetarian Barbecue* by Vicki Rae Chelf and Dominique Biscotti.)

1 pound firm tofu
2 tablespoons plus 1 teaspoon tamari
1 teaspoon toasted sesame oil
1 tablespoon honey
1 teaspoon liquid smoke

3 garlic cloves, pressed
1–2 tablespoons canola oil, as needed,
  plus a little extra for oiling the grid,
  if using a grill

1. Press the water out of the tofu with paper towels and cut it into ¼-inch slices.
2. In a small bowl, combine the tamari, sesame oil, honey, liquid smoke, and garlic; mix well.
3. Brush both sides of the tofu with the liquid mixture and set aside.
4. Prepare the grill or electric grilling machine for cooking.
5. If using a charcoal grill, oil the grid and place it above ashen coals. Brush the tofu lightly with oil and place the slices on the grid directly over the heat. Grill for about 5 minutes, or until nicely browned on the bottom. Brush the tops with oil and turn the slices over. Brush the tops with the tamari mixture and grill for about 5 more minutes. The tofu is done when both sides are nicely browned.
6. If using an electric grilling machine, place the tofu slices on a hot grill and cook for 3 to 5 minutes, or until both sides are nicely browned.
7. Serve with your favorite barbecue sauce in a sandwich or over a bed of brown rice.

Preparation time: *10 minutes*
Cooking time: *about 10 minutes on a grill; 3–5 minutes in an electric grilling machine*
Makes 3–4 servings

Nutritional Breakdown (per serving)

Calories: 125	*Carbohydrates: 9 gm*	*Cholesterol: 0 mg*	*Saturated fat: 1 gm*
Protein: 9 gm	*Sodium: 625 mg*	*Fat: 6 gm*	*% calories fat: 45%*

≋

> Soy products contain substances known as phytoestrogens (plant estrogens) and isoflavonoids (compounds with an estrogenic effect). These plant substances are especially helpful for postmenopausal women with low estrogen levels. A Japanese study of postmenopausal women showed they experienced fewer hot flashes and other symptoms than did Western women. Apparently there is no need to fear an estrogen overload from these plant estrogens, either, because scientists have found that food estrogens desensitize body tissues to this danger.

Vegetarian Kabobs ♡

≋ The sauerkraut lends a German accent to these skewers. Try them on a cool autumn evening for a hearty vegetarian grill. (This recipe is adapted from *The Sensuous Vegetarian Barbecue* by Vicki Rae Chelf and Dominique Biscotti.)

24 small new red potatoes
8 bamboo skewers, soaked in water for
   15–30 minutes
1 large onion, cut into chunks
8 vegetarian hot dogs
4 cups sauerkraut
1 teaspoon caraway seeds

2 tablespoons canola oil plus a little extra
   for the grid, if using a grill
2 tablespoons tamari
1 teaspoon herbes de Provence (see page
   166)
Dijon mustard

1. Scrub the potatoes and steam or pressure-cook them until they just start to get tender. (Be careful not to overcook them or they will fall off the skewers.) Steam the onion pieces until they just start to get tender, 4 to 5 minutes.

2. Cut each hot dog into 3 pieces. Thread the ingredients onto skewers, alternating hot dogs, potatoes, and onion pieces. (If using an electric grilling machine, cut the skewers to fit the machine.)

3. In a small saucepan, mix together the sauerkraut and the caraway seeds, and simmer on low until heated through. Cover and keep warm until needed.

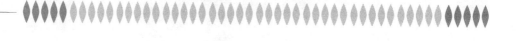

4. In a small bowl, combine the oil, tamari, and herbes de Provence. Brush the oil mixture over the kabobs.

5. Prepare the grill or electric grilling machine for cooking.

6. If using a charcoal grill, oil the grid and place it above ashen coals. Place the kabobs on the coolest part of the grill and cook over indirect heat for about 10 minutes, or until the vegetables are tender and grilled. Turn the kabobs occasionally so they brown evenly and baste with the tamari mixture.

7. If using an electric grilling machine, place as many skewers in the machine as will fit at one time. Cook for 4 to 5 minutes, or until the vegetables are nicely browned and tender.

8. Serve the sauerkraut on individual plates and top with the kabobs. Serve with Dijon mustard.

Preparation time: *25 minutes*
Cooking time: *10 minutes on a grill; 4–5 minutes in an electric grilling machine*
Makes 4 servings (2 kabobs each)

Nutritional Breakdown (per serving)

Calories: 455	*Carbohydrates: 57 gm*	*Cholesterol: 0 mg*	*Saturated fat: 2 gm*
Protein: 29 gm	*Sodium: 2650 mg*	*Fat: 13 gm*	*% calories fat: 25%*

GLOSSARY OF
TERMS AND INGREDIENTS

MOST OF THE RECIPES IN THIS BOOK CONTAIN INGREDIENTS that should be quite familiar. In some cases we do use items or terms you may not recognize. Listed in this section are explanations of ingredients and information on where you should be able to find them, along with some terms that may need to be defined. If you are not familiar with a term or food item that is used in one of our recipes or is recommended as an accompaniment, just look it up here in this section.

Cilantro. Also called Chinese parsley, Mexican parsley, and fresh coriander, cilantro leaves have a bold taste with hints of citrus. Fresh cilantro is available in most grocery stores and Asian markets.

Coconut milk (unsweetened). Unsweetened coconut milk is available in cans and frozen. It can be found at most grocery stores and Asian markets.

Couscous. Of Moroccan origin, couscous is a pasta made from durum wheat, which has more protein than common strains of wheat. Couscous cooks into a light, fluffy consistency and is especially good with lamb. It can be used in place of rice or potatoes and is convenient because it cooks in about 5 minutes. Whole-wheat couscous (the most nutritious) and regular (refined) couscous are available at many grocery stores and health food stores. (Though Cherie and I have not used couscous in any of our recipes, we recommend it as an accompaniment.)

Ginger (fresh). The hot, spicy flavor of this tropical underground plant stem makes it a popular addition to Asian-influenced dishes. Fresh ginger should be peeled before grating or mincing. Ground dried ginger cannot be substituted for fresh ginger in our recipes. Fresh ginger can be found at most grocery stores and Asian markets.

Herbes de Provence. A mixture of herbs that grow plentifully in the south of France, herbes de Provence can be purchased in gourmet and specialty food shops. You can also make your own by combining dried herbs in the following quantities:

3 tablespoons dried thyme
3 tablespoons dried marjoram
3 tablespoons dried summer savory
1 tablespoon dried basil
2 teaspoons dried rosemary
1/2 teaspoon crushed sage
1/2 teaspoon fennel seeds

Mix all the ingredients well and store in a tightly covered glass jar.

Honey. Both sweeter and lighter in calories than white sugar, honey is composed of simple sugars. Its composition, color, and flavor are as varied as the blossoms that attract the bees. The degree of filtering is a factor to consider. Most *raw* honey has been lightly heated and filtered, and retains some enzymes and traces of vitamins and minerals. Most commercial brands have been highly processed. Commercial honey is available in grocery stores, and raw honey is most readily found in health food stores.

Molasses. A by-product of the sugarcane refining process, blackstrap molasses has a strong, bittersweet flavor, while sweet molasses tastes sweeter than blackstrap. (We have used blackstrap in our recipes.) Blackstrap molasses is the final extraction of sugarcane, and it contains calcium, iron, and other minerals. The most nutritious brands are unsulphured and are most readily found at health food stores.

Naturally grown. The label *naturally grown* applies to animals that are raised without added hormones, antibiotics, steroids, or growth stimulants. It also refers to animals that are allowed to roam for their food, rather than being confined to pens at factory farms; the exception is chickens, which are kept in fenced areas rather than in cages. Natural growing practices for beef, lamb, and poultry create healthier animals, which in turn produce healthier food. Meat and poultry labels that say *naturally grown* can be found at many grocery stores and some health food stores, or you can order by mail.

Organically grown. *Organic* refers to the way food is produced. Organic food production is based on a system of farming that maintains and replenishes the fertility of the soil. Organic foods are grown without the use of synthetic pesticides and fertilizers. With healthy soil, plants are better able to resist disease and insects. *Certified organic* means that food has been grown according to strict uniform standards, which are verified by independent state or private organizations.

Roasted peppers. Roast peppers over a gas flame, under a broiler, or on a grill over hot coals. Turn them often until the skin is charred black on all sides. Immediately place the peppers in a paper or plastic bag, seal, and cool for 15 minutes. Then peel off the skin and remove the seeds, stems, and cores.

Tamari. This is a dark brown salty liquid produced from fermented soybeans and used traditionally in Oriental dishes in place of salt. Tamari is preferred over soy sauce, since a modern technique for making soy sauce uses chemical solvents to remove the fat from soybean meal, and adds caramel color and corn syrup for color and flavor along with preservatives. Tamari can be found in many grocery stores and most health food stores.

Thai curry paste. This is an Asian curry paste that comes in red, green, and yellow varieties. It is made from chilies, onion, garlic, spices, and salt. More complex in flavor and hotter in taste than Indian curry paste, it can be found in Asian markets, the international section of many grocery stores, and some health food stores.

Toasted (Asian) sesame oil. This oil is made from toasted sesame seeds and is used primarily for its nutty flavor.

Toasting nuts and seeds. Toasting nuts and seeds brings out their rich flavor, deepens their color, and makes them crunchier. To toast nuts, spread them on a shallow baking pan with edges and place them in a 250° F oven for about 25 to 30 minutes, or until they are golden. Place seeds in a small cast-iron pan in a 250° F oven for 20 minutes, or until golden.

Tofu. A soybean puree, tofu is made by soaking soybeans in water for 8 to 10 hours and then grinding them into a puree. The puree is then pressed through a cloth to extract the soy milk. The milk is cooked and a coagulant (traditionally, nigari) is added to curdle it. The curds are ladled into a mold, where they are pressed until firm. Tofu is stored in cold water. It comes in two textures—soft and firm—and is available at most grocery stores and health food stores.

TVP (textured vegetable [soy] protein). A processed soy product, TVP is in most cases "spun" threads of soy protein that are devoid of taste and aroma. They must be hydrated, and they take on flavors, spices, and colors easily. Mixed with the right ingredients, shaped, and cooked, a product emerges that mimics meat. TVP also can be added to ground meat as an extender and nutrient-enhancer. TVP can most often be found at health food stores.

Vinegar

Balsamic. An Italian wine vinegar aged up to fifty years in wooden barrels. The dark-colored liquid is sweet, smooth, and mellow, and is excellent for marinades as well as salad dressings. Most grocery stores carry balsamic vinegar.

Rice Vinegar. White or brown, this mild-flavored Japanese vinegar comes in seasoned and unseasoned varieties, and is made either from white (refined) or brown rice. White rice vinegar can be found at most grocery stores, and the brown variety at most health food stores.

Zest. This is the flavorful skin of citrus fruits, minus the white pithy part underneath, which is quite bitter. It can be grated or peeled, then minced or cut into julienne. Peel very finely with a sharp knife or a kitchen tool known as a zester.

INDEX

A

Albacore Tuna with Gingered Marinade, 87
apple(s)
    Apple-Cinnamon Sauce, 116
    Kabobs with Sweet Potatoes and, 156–57

B

Barbecued Chicken with Sweet Mustard Sauce,
    118–19
Barbecued Monkfish with Butter-Wine Baste,
    91–92
Barbecued Salmon Fillet with Dill-Wine Baste,
    82–83
Barbecued Sweet Potato–Apple Kabobs,
    156–57
Barbecued Tofu, 162–63
barbecue sauce(s), 42–46
    Cherie's Fat-Free Barbecue Sauce, 46
    LBJ's Texas Barbecue Sauce, 42–43
    Louisiana Bacon, Country-Style Ribs with,
        145–46
    South Carolina Mustard Sauce, 44
    Sweet Vinegar Barbecue Sauce, 45
    Texas, 76–77
barbecuing, described, 31–32

baste(s)
    Butter-Wine, 91–92
    Dill-Wine, Barbecued Salmon Fillet with,
        82–83
    see also marinade(s); dry rub(s)
beef, 63–77
    Cherie's Fat-Free Barbecue Sauce, 46
    Flank Steak Strips with Hot Honey-
        Molasses Sauce, 72–73
    George's Powerburger, 48–49
    George's Sausage Texas-Style, 69–70
    Green Chili and Red Pepper Burgers with
        Roasted Red Pepper Mayonnaise, 49–51
    Grilled Steak and Onion Salad with
        Tarragon-Dijon Dressing, 67–68
    Grilled Steak Strips over Santa Fe Salad,
        65–67
    Grilled Steak with Ginger-Soy Marinade,
        71–72
    Herbed Steak Dijon, 70–71
    LBJ's Texas Barbecue Sauce, 42–43
    Lean, Mean Steak Fajitas, 74–75
    marinades and rubs
        Fat-Free Garlic-Wine Marinade, 34
        Garlic-Herb Rub, 39
        Ginger-Soy Marinade, 36
        John's Hot and Spicy Rub for Ribs, 40

beef (*cont.*)
   Philly Cheese Steak Sandwiches, 57–58
   Texas Barbecued Beef Ribs, 76–77
   tips for handling, 23–24, 64
   see also ribs
benzopyrene, 21
Boneless Chicken Breasts with Fat-Free Garlic-
      Wine Marinade, 122–23
braziers, 26
briquettes, charcoal, 29
Brochettes, Sea Scallop, with Tomato-Yogurt
      Sauce, 95–96
burgers and sandwiches, 47–62
   Cherie's American Gyros with Cucumber-
      Yogurt Sauce, 59–60
   Chicken Burgers with Onion-Dill Sauce,
      52–53
   Deluxe Turkey Burgers, 55–56
   Garden Burgers, 61–62
   George's Powerburger, 48–49
   Green Chili and Red Pepper Burgers with
      Roasted Red Pepper Mayonnaise, 49–51
   Grilled Santa Fe Chicken Burgers, 54–55
   Philly Cheese Steak Sandwiches, 57–58

C

Cajun Spice Rub for Fish, 38
Catfish, George's Fillets with Sesame Crust,
      92–93
The Champ's Sausage Without Guilt, 136–37
charcoal
   briquettes, 29
   hardwood, 30
   lighting, 30–31
   see also grills
Chef Mark's Tomato-Basil Halibut, 85–86
Cherie's American Gyros with Cucumber-
      Yogurt Sauce, 59–60
Cherie's Barbecued Chicken with Apple-
      Cinnamon Sauce, 116–17
Cherie's Fat-Free Barbecue Sauce, 46

chicken, *see* poultry
Chicken Burgers with Onion-Dill Sauce,
      52–53
Chicken Kabobs with Peanut Dipping Sauce,
      126–27
Chicken Parmesan, Grilled, 121–22
chili peppers
   Green Chili and Red Pepper Burgers with
      Roasted Red Pepper Mayonnaise, 49–51
   South of the Border Salsa, 66
Country-Style Ribs with Louisiana Bacon
      Barbecue Sauce, 145–46
Cucumber-Yogurt Sauce, 59–60

D

Deluxe Turkey Burgers, 55–56
docosahexaenoic acid (DHA), 11
dry rub(s), 37–41
   Cajun Spice Rub for Fish, 38
   Dill-Wine Dry Rub, 89–90
   Garlic-Herb Rub, 39
   John's Hot and Spicy Rub for Ribs, 40
   Spice and Herb Rub for Lamb, 41
   Thyme–Bay Leaf Rub, 37–38
   see also baste(s); marinade(s)

E

E. coli, 21, 23–24
eicosapentaenoic acid (EPA), 11

F

Fajitas, Lean, Mean Steak, 74–75
fat, 9–11
   artificial, 10
   beneficial, 10–11
   in Food Guide Pyramid, 13, 15
   tips for reducing, 22–23

fat-free foods
  Barbecue Sauce, Cherie's, 46
  dangers of, 10
  Garlic-Wine Marinade, 34, 122–23
  Zesty Fat-Free Marinade, 33–34
fire lighters, 30–31
fish and seafood, 78–98
  Albacore Tuna with Gingered Marinade, 87
  Barbecued Monkfish with Butter-Wine
    Baste, 91–92
  Barbecued Salmon Fillet with Dill-Wine
    Baste, 82–83
  Chef Mark's Tomato-Basil Halibut, 85–86
  George's Catfish Fillets with Sesame Crust,
    92–93
  Ginger-Lime Swordfish, 83–84
  Grilled Flounder with Dill-Wine Dry Rub,
    89–90
  Grilled Salmon Steaks with Tarragon Sauce,
    80–81
  marinades and rubs
    Cajun Spice Rub for, 38
    Raspberry Vinegar Marinade, 35–36
    Rosemary-Thyme Marinade, 35
    Thyme–Bay Leaf Rub, 37–38
    Zesty Fat-Free Marinade, 33–34
  omega fatty acids in, 11
  Orange Roughy with Zesty Fat-Free
    Marinade, 88–89
  Sea Scallop Brochettes with Tomato-Yogurt
    Sauce, 95–96
  Sweet Vinegar Barbecue Sauce, 45
  Thai Shrimp Kabobs, 97–98
  tips for handling, 23–24, 79
  Zesty Citrus-Thyme Shrimp Kabobs, 93–94
Flank Steak Strips with Hot Honey-Molasses
  Sauce, 72–73
Flounder, Grilled, with Dill-Wine Dry Rub,
  89–90
Food Guide Pyramid, 12–15
food poisoning, 23–24
The Foreman Family Breakfast Sausage, 140
fruits, in Food Guide Pyramid, 13, 14

G

gamma-linoleic acid (GLA), 11
Garden Burgers, 61–62
garlic
  and cholesterol, 23
  Fat-Free Marinade with Wine and, 34
  Garlic-Herb Rub, 39
  and HCAs, 21
  Roasted, 159–60
George's Catfish Fillets with Sesame Crust,
  92–93
George's Powerburger, 48–49
George's Sausage Texas-Style, 69–70
Ginger-Lime Swordfish, 83–84
Ginger Pork Salad, 151–52
Ginger-Soy Marinade, 36, 71–72
Green Chili and Red Pepper Burgers with
  Roasted Red Pepper Mayonnaise, 49–51
Grilled Chicken Parmesan, 121–22
Grilled Chicken Thighs over Acapulco Salad,
  128–29
Grilled Flounder with Dill-Wine Dry Rub,
  89–90
Grilled Lamb Chops with Plum Sauce, 110–11
Grilled Lamb Salad with Hot Minted-Wine
  Dressing, 101–2
Grilled Pork Chops with Sage-Wine Marinade,
  143–44
Grilled Salmon Steaks with Tarragon Sauce,
  80–81
Grilled Santa Fe Chicken Burgers, 54–55
Grilled Steak and Onion Salad with Tarragon-
  Dijon Dressing, 67–68
Grilled Steak Strips over Santa Fe Salad, 65–67
Grilled Steak with Ginger-Soy Marinade, 71–72
Grilled Turkey Cutlets with Honey-Dijon-
  Rosemary Marinade, 134–35
grilling
  cooking times for, 32
  described, 31
  tips for, 21–22, 64, 79, 100, 113, 139
  see also specific types of food

grills, 25–32
  accessories for, 27–29
  electric, 27
  fire starters, 30–31
  gas, 26–27
  kettle-shaped, 26
  lighting, 29–31
  open, 26
  outdoor cooking methods, 31–32
  rectangular hinged, 26

H

Halibut, Chef Mark's Tomato-Basil, 85–86
hardwood charcoal, 30
hardwood chips, chunks, and sawdust, 30
Herbed Steak Dijon, 70–71
heterocyclic amines (HCAs), 21

J

Joan's Rosemary Lamb Chops, 107–8
John's Hot and Spicy Rub for Ribs, 40

K

kabob(s)
  Barbecued Sweet Potato–Apple, 156–57
  Chicken, with Peanut Dipping Sauce,
    126–27
  Shish Kabobs with Fresh Mint Marinade,
    103–4
  Shrimp, Thai, 97–98
  Shrimp, Zesty Citrus-Thyme, 93–94
  Vegetable, with Raspberry Vinegar
    Marinade, 155
  Vegetarian, 163–64
kindling, 30
Knock-Out-the-Fat Tacos, 133–34

L

lamb, 99–111
  Cherie's American Gyros with Cucumber-
    Yogurt Sauce, 59–60
  Grilled Lamb Chops with Plum Sauce,
    110–11
  Grilled Lamb Salad with Hot Minted-Wine
    Dressing, 101–2
  Joan's Rosemary Lamb Chops, 107–8
  Lamb Chops with Minted Tomato Salsa,
    105–6
  marinades and rubs
    Garlic-Herb Rub, 39
    Spice and Herb Rub for, 41
  Shish Kabobs with Fresh Mint Marinade,
    103–4
  Spice-and-Herb-Crusted Lamb with Yogurt
    Sauce, 108–9
  tips for handling, 23–24, 100
LBJ's Texas Barbecue Sauce, 42–43
Lean, Mean Steak Fajitas, 74–75
lighter fluid, 30–31
linoleic acid, 11

M

marinade(s), 33–36
  Balsamic, Mixed Vegetable Grill with,
    157–58
  Fat-Free Garlic-Wine, 34, 122–23
  Fresh Basil-Balsamic Vinegar, 121
  Fresh Mint, 103
  Gingered, 87
  Ginger-Lime, 83–84
  Ginger-Sesame, 149–50
  Ginger-Soy, 36, 71–72
  Honey-Dijon-Rosemary, 134–35
  Honey-Pineapple, 141–43
  Mint, 101–2
  Raspberry Vinegar, 35–36, 155
  Rosemary, 107
  Rosemary-Thyme, 35

Sage-Wine, 143–44
Tomato-Basil, 85–86
Zesty Fat-Free, 33–34, 88–89
see also baste(s); dry rub(s)
mayonnaise, 22
Roasted Red Pepper, 51
mesquite charcoal, 30
Mixed Vegetable Grill with Balsamic Marinade, 157–58
Monkfish, Barbecued, with Butter-Wine Baste, 91–92
Mustard Sauce, South Carolina, 44

O

omega fatty acids, 11
onion(s)
and cholesterol, 23
Grilled Steak and Onion Salad with Tarragon-Dill Dressing, 67–68
Onion-Dill Sauce, 53
Orange Roughy with Zesty Fat-Free Marinade, 88–89

P

peppers
Green Chili and Red Pepper Burgers with Roasted Red Pepper Mayonnaise, 49–51
Roasted Red, 160–61
see also chili peppers
Philly Cheese Steak Sandwiches, 57–58
Plum Sauce, 110–11
polycyclic aromatic carbons (PAHs), 21
pork, 138–52
Country-Style Ribs with Louisiana Bacon Barbecue Sauce, 145–46
The Foreman Family Breakfast Sausage, 140
Ginger Pork Salad, 151–52
Grilled Pork Chops with Sage-Wine Marinade, 143–44
John's Hot and Spicy Rub for Ribs, 40

LBJ's Texas Barbecue Sauce, 42–43
Pork and Pineapple Skewers with Ginger-Sesame Marinade, 149–50
South Carolina Mustard Sauce, 44
Southeast Asian Spareribs, 147–48
Stuffed Pork Chops with Honey-Pineapple Marinade, 141–43
tips for handling, 23–24, 139
see also ribs
Potatoes, Roasted New, with Garlic and Rosemary, 158–59
poultry, 112–37
Barbecued Chicken with Sweet Mustard Sauce, 118–19
Boneless Chicken Breasts with Fat-Free Garlic-Wine Marinade, 122–23
The Champ's Sausage Without Guilt, 136–37
Cherie's Barbecued Chicken with Apple-Cinnamon Sauce, 116–17
Cherie's Fat-Free Barbecue Sauce, 46
Chicken Burgers with Onion-Dill Sauce, 52–53
Chicken Kabobs with Peanut Dipping Sauce, 126–27
Deluxe Turkey Burgers, 55–56
Grilled Chicken Parmesan, 121–22
Grilled Chicken Thighs over Acapulco Salad, 128–29
Grilled Santa Fe Chicken Burgers, 54–55
Grilled Turkey Cutlets with Honey-Dijon-Rosemary Marinade, 134–35
Knock-Out-the-Fat Tacos, 133–34
marinades and rubs
Fat-Free Garlic-Wine Marinade, 34
Ginger-Soy Marinade, 36
Raspberry Vinegar Marinade, 35–36
Rosemary-Thyme Marinade, 35
Zesty Fat-Free Marinade, 33–34
Ranch-Style Honey Barbecued Chicken, 114–15
Rosemary-Thyme Chicken Strips over Lemon-Garlic Caesar Salad, 130–32
South Carolina Mustard Sauce, 44

poultry (*cont.*)

    Stuffed Chicken Breasts with Peach-Pecan Stuffing, 123–25

    Sweet Vinegar Barbecue Sauce, 45

    Texas Cowboy BBQ Drumsticks, 119–20

    tips for handling, 23–24, 55, 113, 120

R

Ranch-Style Honey Barbecued Chicken, 114–15

Raspberry Vinegar Marinade, 35–36

red peppers

    Mayonnaise with Roasted, 51

    Roasted, 160–61

ribs

    Country-Style, with Louisiana Bacon Barbecue Sauce, 145–46

    John's Hot and Spicy Rub for, 40

    LBJ's Texas Barbecue Sauce, 42–43

    South Carolina Mustard Sauce, 44

    Southeast Asian Spareribs, 147–48

    Texas Barbecued Beef, 76–77

Roasted Garlic, 159–60

Roasted New Potatoes with Garlic and Rosemary, 158–59

Roasted Red Peppers, 160–61

Rosemary Lamb Chops, Joan's, 107–8

Rosemary-Thyme Chicken Strips over Lemon-Garlic Caesar Salad, 130–32

Rosemary-Thyme Marinade, 35

Roughy, Orange, with Zesty Fat-Free Marinade, 88–89

rubs, *see* dry rub(s)

S

salad(s)

    Acapulco, Grilled Chicken Thighs over, 128–29

    Caesar, Rosemary-Thyme Chicken Strips over Lemon-Garlic, 130–32

Ginger Pork, 151–52

Grilled Lamb, with Hot Minted-Wine Dressing, 101–2

Grilled Steak and Onion, with Tarragon-Dijon Dressing, 67–68

Santa Fe, Grilled Steak Strips over, 65–67

salmon

    Barbecued Fillet with Dill-Wine Baste, 82–83

    Grilled Steaks with Tarragon Sauce, 80–81

salmonella, 23–24

salsa

    Minted Tomato, 105–6

    South of the Border, 66

sandwiches, *see* burgers and sandwiches

sauce(s)

    Apple-Cinnamon, 116

    Cilantro Sour Cream, 133

    Cucumber-Yogurt, 59–60

    Honey Barbecue, 114

    Hot Honey-Molasses, 72–73

    Onion-Dill, 53

    Peanut, 126, 127

    Plum, 110–11

    Sweet Mustard, 118

    Tarragon, 80–81

    Tomato-Yogurt, 95–96

    vegetable, 57–58

    Yogurt, 108–9

    see also barbecue sauce(s)

sausage(s)

    The Champ's, Without Guilt, 136–37

    The Foreman Family Breakfast, 140

    George's Sausage Texas-Style, 69–70

seafood, *see* fish and seafood

Sea Scallop Brochettes with Tomato-Yogurt Sauce, 95–96

Sesame Crust, George's Catfish Fillets with, 92–93

Shish Kabobs with Fresh Mint Marinade, 103–4

shrimp

    Thai Shrimp Kabobs, 97–98

    Zesty Citrus-Thyme Kabobs, 93–94

South Carolina Mustard Sauce, 44
Southeast Asian Spareribs, 147–48
South of the Border Salsa, 66
Spareribs, Southeast Asian, 147–48
Spice-and-Herb-Crusted Lamb with Yogurt
        Sauce, 108–9
Spice and Herb Rub for Lamb, 41
Steak Dijon, Herbed, 70–71
Stuffed Chicken Breasts with Peach-Pecan
        Stuffing, 123–25
Stuffed Pork Chops with Honey-Pineapple
        Marinade, 141–43
Sweet Potatoes, Kabobs with Apples and, 156–57
Sweet Vinegar Barbecue Sauce, 45
Swordfish, Ginger-Lime, 83–84

T

Tacos, Knock-Out-the-Fat, 133–34
Texas Barbecued Beef Ribs, 76–77
Texas Cowboy BBQ Drumsticks, 119–20
textured vegetable (soy) protein (TVP), 21
Thai Shrimp Kabobs, 97–98
Thyme–Bay Leaf Rub, 37–38
Tofu, Barbecued, 162–63
tomato(es)
    Chef Mark's Tomato-Basil Halibut, 85–86
    Minted Tomato Salsa, 105–6
    Sea Scallop Brochettes with Tomato-Yogurt
        Sauce, 95–96
    South of the Border Salsa, 66
Tuna, Albacore, with Gingered Marinade, 87
turkey, *see* poultry

V

vegetables, 153–64
    Barbecued Sweet Potato–Apple Kabobs,
        156–57
    Barbecued Tofu, 162–63
    in Food Guide Pyramid, 12–14
    Garden Burgers, 61–62
    Kabobs with Raspberry Vinegar Marinade,
        155
    Mixed Vegetable Grill with Balsamic
        Marinade, 157–58
    Raspberry Vinegar Marinade, 35–36
    Roasted Garlic, 159–60
    Roasted New Potatoes with Garlic and
        Rosemary, 158–59
    Roasted Red Peppers, 160–61
    tips for handling, 50, 154
    Vegetarian Kabobs, 163–64

Y

yogurt, 22
    Cucumber-Yogurt Sauce, 59–60
    Onion-Dill Sauce, 53
    Sauce, 108–9

Z

Zesty Citrus-Thyme Shrimp Kabobs, 93–94
Zesty Fat-Free Marinade, 33–34

ABOUT THE AUTHORS

GEORGE FOREMAN has twice been the heavyweight champion of the world and is the author of *By George*, published by Villard Books in 1995. He lives in Kingwood, Texas.

Known as a leading expert in nutrition, CHERIE CALBOM, M.S., C.N., is a certified nutritionist and co-author of the bestselling book *Juicing for Life*, and author of *The Healthy Gourmet*, published in February 1996.

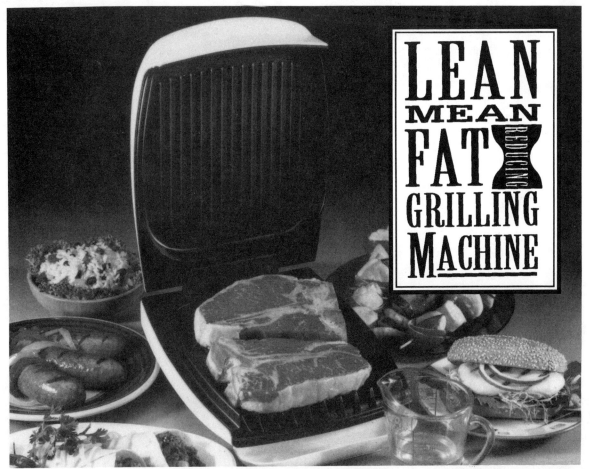

The *George Foreman* LEAN, MEAN FAT REDUCING GRILLING MACHINE

— The very best indoor grill!

Here's why:

- Patented technology that sears in the flavors and channels the fat away from your food at the same time!

- Innovative design with a floating hinge system so foods are cooked from both sides evenly! From stuffed pork chops to fajitas.

- Non-stop, continuous even grilling — thermostat controlled.

- Large cooking surface, holds 4 chicken breasts, 4 big burgers or 2 good-sized steaks at a time.

- Incredibly easy to clean! This grill takes seconds to wipe off with a damp sponge or paper towels.

  Once you see how easy it is to clean, you'll use it every day!

- Double coated non-stick surface for durability and long lasting wear.

PLUS with your **LEAN, MEAN FAT REDUCING GRILLING MACHINE** order, you'll also get:

- Video Recipe Guide featuring Cherie Calbom.
- Taco/Fajita Kit
- LEAN, MEAN DEFROSTING TRAY Thaws out steaks in minutes.

ALL THIS FOR ONLY $89.85 plus $9.95 **Shipping & Handling**

To order this great package, call now!

1-800-800-8455

or send check/money order to: Salton/Maxim Housewares, P.O. Box 473, Louisiana, MO 63353